POISONS
AND
TOXINS

GENERAL EDITORS

Dale C. Garell, M.D.
Medical Director, California Children Services, Department of Health Services,
    County of Los Angeles
Associate Dean for Curriculum; Clinical Professor, Department of Pediatrics &
    Family Medicine, University of Southern California School of Medicine
Former President, Society for Adolescent Medicine

Solomon H. Snyder, M.D.
Distinguished Service Professor of Neuroscience, Pharmacology, and Psychiatry,
    Johns Hopkins University School of Medicine
Former President, Society for Neuroscience
Albert Lasker Award in Medical Research, 1978

CONSULTING EDITORS

Robert W. Blum, M.D., Ph.D.
Professor and Director, Division of General Pediatrics and Adolescent Health,
    University of Minnesota

Charles E. Irwin, Jr., M.D.
Professor of Pediatrics; Director, Division of Adolescent Medicine, University of
    California, San Francisco

Lloyd J. Kolbe, Ph.D.
Director of the Division of Adolescent and School Health, Center for Chronic
    Disease Prevention and Health Promotion, Centers for Disease Control

Jordan J. Popkin
Former Director, Division of Federal Employee Occupational Health, U.S. Public
    Health Service Region I

Joseph L. Rauh, M.D.
Professor of Pediatrics and Medicine, Adolescent Medicine, Children's Hospital
    Medical Center, Cincinnati
Former President, Society for Adolescent Medicine

THE ENCYCLOPEDIA OF
H E A L T H

MEDICAL DISORDERS
AND THEIR TREATMENT

Dale C. Garell, M.D. · General Editor

POISONS
AND
TOXINS

Marc Kusinitz

Introduction by C. Everett Koop, M.D., Sc.D.
former Surgeon General, U. S. Public Health Service

CHELSEA HOUSE PUBLISHERS
New York · Philadelphia

The goal of the ENCYCLOPEDIA OF HEALTH *is to provide general information in the ever-changing areas of physiology, psychology, and related medical issues. The titles in this series are not intended to take the place of the professional advice of a physician or other health care professional.*

ON THE COVER   *Escherichia Coli* bacteria dividing. *E. Coli* is one of the prominent bacteria in the intestinal tract. Color enhanced and magnified 21,000 times.

CHELSEA HOUSE PUBLISHERS
EDITOR-IN-CHIEF   Richard S. Papale
MANAGING EDITOR   Karyn Gullen Browne
COPY CHIEF   Philip Koslow
PICTURE EDITOR   Adrian G. Allen
MANUFACTURING DIRECTOR   Gerald Levine
SYSTEMS MANAGER   Lindsey Ottman
PRODUCTION COORDINATOR   Marie Claire Cebrián-Ume

The Encyclopedia of Health
SENIOR EDITOR   Kenneth W. Lane

Staff for POISONS AND TOXINS
COPY EDITOR   David Carter
EDITORIAL ASSISTANT   Laura Petermann
PICTURE RESEARCHER   Toby Greenberg
DESIGNER   Robert Yaffe

First Printing
1   3   5   7   9   8   6   4   2

Library of Congress Cataloging-in-Publication Data

Kusinitz, Marc
   Poisons and toxins/by Marc Kusinitz; introduction by C. Everett Koop.
      p. cm.—(The Encyclopedia of health)
   Includes bibliographical references and index.
   Summary: Examines the various types of poisons and toxins, their sources, and their effect on the human body.
   ISBN 0-7910-0074-5
         0-7910-0501-1 (pbk.)
   1. Toxins—Juvenile literature. 2. Poisons—Juvenile literature. [1. Poisons. 2. Toxins.] I. Title. II. Series.   92-5967
QP631.K87 1992   CIP
615.9—dc20   AC

CONTENTS

THE ENCYCLOPEDIA OF
H E A L T H

THE HEALTHY BODY

The Circulatory System
Dental Health
The Digestive System
The Endocrine System
Exercise
Genetics & Heredity
The Human Body: An Overview
Hygiene
The Immune System
Memory & Learning
The Musculoskeletal System
The Nervous System
Nutrition
The Reproductive System
The Respiratory System
The Senses
Sleep
Speech & Hearing
Sports Medicine
Vision
Vitamins & Minerals

THE LIFE CYCLE

Adolescence
Adulthood
Aging
Childhood
Death & Dying
The Family
Friendship & Love
Pregnancy & Birth

MEDICAL ISSUES

Careers in Health Care
Environmental Health
Folk Medicine
Health Care Delivery
Holistic Medicine
Medical Ethics
Medical Fakes & Frauds
Medical Technology
Medicine & the Law
Occupational Health
Public Health

PSYCHOLOGICAL DISORDERS AND THEIR TREATMENT

Anxiety & Phobias
Child Abuse
Compulsive Behavior
Delinquency & Criminal Behavior
Depression
Diagnosing & Treating Mental Illness
Eating Habits & Disorders
Learning Disabilities
Mental Retardation
Personality Disorders
Schizophrenia
Stress Management
Suicide

MEDICAL DISORDERS AND THEIR TREATMENT

AIDS
Allergies
Alzheimer's Disease
Arthritis
Birth Defects
Cancer
The Common Cold
Diabetes
Emergency Medicine
Gynecological Disorders
Headaches
The Hospital
Kidney Disorders
Medical Diagnosis
The Mind-Body Connection
Mononucleosis and Other Infectious Diseases
Nuclear Medicine
Organ Transplants
Pain
Physical Handicaps
Poisons & Toxins
Prescription & OTC Drugs
Sexually Transmitted Diseases
Skin Disorders
Stroke & Heart Disease
Substance Abuse
Tropical Medicine

PREVENTION AND EDUCATION: THE KEYS TO GOOD HEALTH

C. Everett Koop, M.D., Sc.D.
former Surgeon General,
U.S. Public Health Service

The issue of health education has received particular attention in recent years because of the presence of AIDS in the news. But our response to this particular tragedy points up a number of broader issues that doctors, public health officials, educators, and the public face. In particular, it points up the necessity for sound health education for citizens of all ages.

Over the past 25 years this country has been able to bring about dramatic declines in the death rates for heart disease, stroke, accidents, and for people under the age of 45, cancer. Today, Americans generally eat better and take better care of themselves than ever before. Thus, with the help of modern science and technology, they have a better chance of surviving serious—even catastrophic—illnesses. That's the good news.

But, like every phonograph record, there's a flip side, and one with special significance for young adults. According to a report issued in 1979 by Dr. Julius Richmond, my predecessor as Surgeon General, Americans aged 15 to 24 had a higher death rate in 1979 than they did 20 years earlier. The causes: violent death and injury, alcohol and drug abuse, unwanted pregnancies, and sexually transmitted diseases. Adolescents are particularly vulnerable because they are beginning to explore their own sexuality and perhaps to experiment with drugs. The need for educating young people is critical, and the price of neglect is high.

Yet even for the population as a whole, our health is still far from what it could be. Why? A 1974 Canadian government report attributed all death and disease to four broad elements: inadequacies in the health care system, behavioral factors or unhealthy life-styles, environmental hazards, and human biological factors.

To be sure, there are diseases that are still beyond the control of even our advanced medical knowledge and techniques. And despite yearnings that are as old as the human race itself, there is no "fountain of youth" to ward off aging and death. Still, there is a solution to many of the problems that undermine sound health. In a word, that solution is prevention. Prevention, which includes health promotion and education, saves lives, improves the quality of life, and in the long run, saves money.

In the United States, organized public health activities and preventive medicine have a long history. Important milestones in this country or foreign breakthroughs adopted in the United States include the improvement of sanitary procedures and the development of pasteurized milk in the late 19th century and the introduction in the mid-20th century of effective vaccines against polio, measles, German measles, mumps, and other once-rampant diseases. Internationally, organized public health efforts began on a wide-scale basis with the International Sanitary Conference of 1851, to which 12 nations sent representatives. The World Health Organization, founded in 1948, continues these efforts under the aegis of the United Nations, with particular emphasis on combating communicable diseases and the training of health care workers.

Despite these accomplishments, much remains to be done in the field of prevention. For too long, we have had a medical care system that is science- and technology-based, focused, essentially, on illness and mortality. It is now patently obvious that both the social and the economic costs of such a system are becoming insupportable.

Implementing prevention—and its corollaries, health education and promotion—is the job of several groups of people.

First, the medical and scientific professions need to continue basic scientific research, and here we are making considerable progress. But increased concern with prevention will also have a decided impact on how primary care doctors practice medicine. With a shift to health-based rather than morbidity-based medicine, the role of the "new physician" will include a healthy dose of patient education.

Second, practitioners of the social and behavioral sciences— psychologists, economists, city planners—along with lawyers, business leaders, and government officials—must solve the practical and ethical dilemmas confronting us: poverty, crime, civil rights, literacy, education, employment, housing, sanitation, environmental protection, health care delivery systems, and so forth. All of these issues affect public health.

Third is the public at large. We'll consider that very important group in a moment.

Fourth, and the linchpin in this effort, is the public health profession—doctors, epidemiologists, teachers—who must harness the professional expertise of the first two groups and the common sense and cooperation of the third, the public. They must define the problems statistically and qualitatively and then help us set priorities for finding the solutions.

To a very large extent, improving those statistics is the responsibility of every individual. So let's consider more specifically what the role of the individual should be and why health education is so important to that role. First, and most obvious, individuals can protect themselves from illness and injury and thus minimize their need for professional medical care. They can eat nutritious food; get adequate exercise; avoid tobacco, alcohol, and drugs; and take prudent steps to avoid accidents. The proverbial "apple a day keeps the doctor away" is not so far from the truth, after all.

Second, individuals should actively participate in their own medical care. They should schedule regular medical and dental checkups. Should they develop an illness or injury, they should know when to treat themselves and when to seek professional help. To gain the maximum benefit from any medical treatment that they do require, individuals must become partners in that treatment. For instance, they should understand the effects and side effects of medications. I counsel young physicians that there is no such thing as too much information when talking with patients. But the corollary is the patient must know enough about the nuts and bolts of the healing process to understand what the doctor is telling him or her. That is at least partially the patient's responsibility.

Education is equally necessary for us to understand the ethical and public policy issues in health care today. Sometimes individuals will encounter these issues in making decisions about their own treatment or that of family members. Other citizens may encounter them as jurors in medical malpractice cases. But we all become involved, indirectly, when we elect our public officials, from school board members to the president. Should surrogate parenting be legal? To what extent is drug testing desirable, legal, or necessary? Should there be public funding for family planning, hospitals, various types of medical research, and other medical care for the indigent? How should we allocate scant technological resources, such as kidney dialysis and organ transplants? What is the proper role of government in protecting the rights of patients?

What are the broad goals of public health in the United States today? In 1980, the Public Health Service issued a report aptly entitled *Promoting Health—Preventing Disease: Objectives for the Nation*. This report expressed its goals in terms of mortality and in terms of intermediate goals in education and health improvement. It identified 15 major concerns: controlling high blood pressure; improving family planning; improving pregnancy care and infant health; increasing the rate of immunization; controlling sexually transmitted diseases; controlling the presence of toxic agents and radiation in the environment; improving occupational safety and health; preventing accidents; promoting water fluoridation and dental health; controlling infectious diseases; decreasing smoking; decreasing alcohol and drug abuse; improving nutrition; promoting physical fitness and exercise; and controlling stress and violent behavior.

For healthy adolescents and young adults (ages 15 to 24), the specific goal was a 20% reduction in deaths, with a special focus on motor vehicle injuries and alcohol and drug abuse. For adults (ages 25 to 64), the aim was 25% fewer deaths, with a concentration on heart attacks, strokes, and cancers.

Smoking is perhaps the best example of how individual behavior can have a direct impact on health. Today, cigarette smoking is recognized as the single most important preventable cause of death in our society. It is responsible for more cancers and more cancer deaths than any other known agent; is a prime risk factor for heart and blood vessel disease, chronic bronchitis, and emphysema; and is a frequent cause of complications in pregnancies and of babies born prematurely, underweight, or with potentially fatal respiratory and cardiovascular problems.

Since the release of the Surgeon General's first report on smoking in 1964, the proportion of adult smokers has declined substantially, from 43% in 1965 to 30.5% in 1985. Since 1965, 37 million people have quit smoking. Although there is still much work to be done if we are to become a "smoke-free society," it is heartening to note that public health and public education efforts—such as warnings on cigarette packages and bans on broadcast advertising—have already had significant effects.

In 1835, Alexis de Tocqueville, a French visitor to America, wrote, "In America the passion for physical well-being is general." Today, as then, health and fitness are front-page items. But with the greater scientific and technological resources now available to us, we are in a far stronger position to make good health care available to everyone. And with the greater technological threats to us as we approach the 21st century, the need to do so is more urgent than ever before. Comprehensive information about basic biology, preventive medicine, medical and surgical treatments, and related ethical and public policy issues can help you arm yourself with the knowledge you need to be healthy throughout your life.

FOREWORD

Dale C. Garell, M.D.

Advances in our understanding of health and disease during the 20th century have been truly remarkable. Indeed, it could be argued that modern health care is one of the greatest accomplishments in all of human history. In the early 20th century, improvements in sanitation, water treatment, and sewage disposal reduced death rates and increased longevity. Previously untreatable illnesses can now be managed with antibiotics, immunizations, and modern surgical techniques. Discoveries in the fields of immunology, genetic diagnosis, and organ transplantation are revolutionizing the prevention and treatment of disease. Modern medicine is even making inroads against cancer and heart disease, two of the leading causes of death in the United States.

Although there is much to be proud of, medicine continues to face enormous challenges. Science has vanquished diseases such as smallpox and polio, but new killers, most notably AIDS, confront us. Moreover, we now victimize ourselves with what some have called "diseases of choice," or those brought on by drug and alcohol abuse, bad eating habits, and mismanagement of the stresses and strains of contemporary life. The very technology that is doing so much to prolong life has brought with it previously unimaginable ethical dilemmas related to issues of death and dying. The rising cost of health care is a matter of central concern to us all. And violence in the form of automobile accidents, homicide, and suicide remains the major killer of young adults.

In the past, most people were content to leave health care and medical treatment in the hands of professionals. But since the 1960s, the consumer of medical care—that is, the patient—has assumed an increasingly central role in the management of his or her own health. There has also been a new emphasis placed on prevention: People are recognizing that their own actions can help prevent many of the conditions that have caused death and disease in the past. This accounts for the growing commitment to good nutrition and regular exercise, for the increasing number of people who are choosing not to smoke, and for a new moderation in people's drinking habits.

People want to know more about themselves and their own health. They are curious about their body: its anatomy, physiology, and biochemistry. They want to keep up with rapidly evolving medical technologies and procedures. They are willing to educate themselves about common disorders and diseases so that they can be full partners in their own health care.

THE ENCYCLOPEDIA OF HEALTH is designed to provide the basic knowledge that readers will need if they are to take significant responsibility for their own health. It is also meant to serve as a frame of reference for further study and exploration. The encyclopedia is divided into five subsections: The Healthy Body; The Life Cycle; Medical Disorders & Their Treatment; Psychological Disorders & Their Treatment; and Medical Issues. For each topic covered by the encyclopedia, we present the essential facts about the relevant biology; the symptoms, diagnosis, and treatment of common diseases and disorders; and ways in which you can prevent or reduce the severity of health problems when that is possible. The encyclopedia also projects what may lie ahead in the way of future treatment or prevention strategies.

The broad range of topics and issues covered in the encyclopedia reflects that human health encompasses physical, psychological, social, environmental, and spiritual well-being. Just as the mind and the body are inextricably linked, so, too, is the individual an integral part of the wider world that comprises his or her family, society, and environment. To discuss health in its broadest aspect it is necessary to explore the many ways in which it is connected to such fields as law, social science, public policy, economics, and even religion. And so, the encyclopedia is meant to be a bridge between science, medical technology, the world at large, and you. I hope that it will inspire you to pursue in greater depth particular areas of interest and that you will take advantage of the suggestions for further reading and the lists of resources and organizations that can provide additional information.

CHAPTER 1

POISON PRIMER

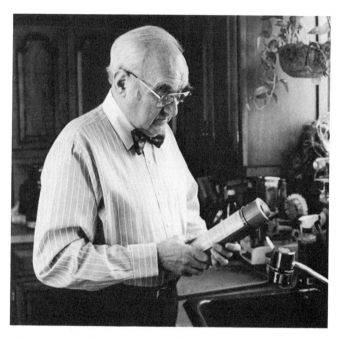

When purchasing a potentially dangerous product, it is essential to read the label carefully. This will help the purchaser to determine how toxic the substance is and what to do in case poisoning should occur.

A *poison* is any substance that, once inside the body, produces harmful chemical reactions that interfere with the body's normal functions. A *toxin* is a poison that comes from a plant or animal. For example, poison injected from a snakebite is considered a toxin, but harmful substances found in car exhaust are not. Theoretically, if the amount consumed is great enough, just about anything can be poisonous.

A report by the American Association of Poison Control Centers (AAPCC) examined poisoning reports for the year 1990, using data from 72 poison centers that participated in the study. Although not every center in the country took part in the survey, those that did served an area covering the majority of the United States. Among the participating centers alone, more than 1.7 million cases of human exposure to poison were reported, and it was estimated that more than 2.2 million exposures were reported to all poison control centers that year. Of course, these figures just refer to *reported* poisonings as opposed to *actual* poisonings. In many of these cases, the individual who was reported to the center may not have been poisoned at all, but instead may have ingested something harmless that he or she simply thought was dangerous. The AAPCC study did not estimate the number of actual poisonings in the United States.

The annual number of poison-related deaths that occur each year is also difficult to gauge. The AAPCC study, for example, found 612 reported fatalities in 1990. But according to the *Handbook of Poisoning: Prevention, Diagnosis, & Treatment,* by Robert H. Dreisbach and William O. Robertson, more than 12,000 poison-related deaths are believed to occur each year in the United States.

SUICIDE

Poisonings don't always occur by accident, either. Although no one knows exactly how many suicidal poisonings occur each year, the National Center for Health Statistics of the Centers for Disease Control has determined that in 1988 alone (the latest year for such figures), 351 young people between the ages of 10 and 19 years took their lives by taking overdoses of drugs or other substances.

Among teenagers aged 15 to 19, 137 individuals used drugs to commit suicide; 183 used some sort of gas or vapor, such as automobile exhaust; and 10 used a solid or liquid substance, such as a pesticide, corrosive chemical, or compound containing arsenic. And while no child aged 10 to 14 years was reported to have committed suicide by taking such solid or liquid substances, 16 children in this age group did take overdoses of drugs, and 5 died by inhaling poisonous gases.

According to the Report of the Secretary's Task Force on Youth Suicide, there is a link between suicidal behavior and substance abuse in adolescents.

Among heavy substance abusers, there is a fourfold greater suicidal death rate than in the rest of the population. The report also cites a 1972 study (*The Lancet*) showing that among adolescents 12 to 19 years old, 41% of the boys and 19% of the girls had been drinking immediately before attempting suicide.

Why is poisoning such a common occurrence? One reason may be the large number of *toxic* (poisonous) substances that lurk in familiar places. Drugs in the family medicine cabinet can be abused. Lead in the pipes of water supply systems threaten the health of consumers and the physical and mental development of children. Food, if it is improperly prepared or stored, is vulnerable to contamination. Even the family car spews deadly *carbon monoxide*—odorless and invisible—which can kill in minutes. According to the AAPCC, cleaning substances (180,096 of them) were the most prevalent source of reported poisonings in 1990 (although only 26 were known to result in death).

Medical authorities have warned the federal government that increasing numbers of Americans are falling ill from exposure to popular

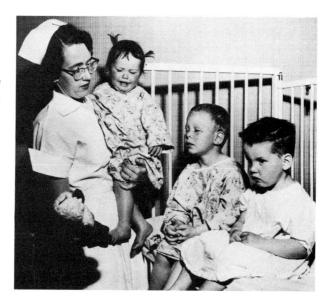

A 1957 news photo of three children treated at a California hospital; the youngsters ate rat poison, which they had mistaken for breakfast cereal.

lawn and garden pesticides. Yet almost none of these chemicals have been fully evaluated for their safety, according to the U.S. Environmental Protection Agency (EPA). The EPA estimates that about 45,000 people annually report accidental pesticide poisonings.

In many instances, however, tragedy can be avoided. Despite the wide variety of potentially deadly substances found in the home and workplace, some straightforward measures can prevent poisoning or save the life of someone who has been exposed to a toxic substance.

PREVENTION

The key word in poison prevention is *care*. It is essential to buy potentially dangerous products with care, use them with care, and store them with care.

Poisonous Products

Before buying a product that is toxic, a consumer should remember three rules:

- *Read the label* on the container to make sure that the product has been made for the desired use.

- *Buy the least hazardous product* capable of performing the required job. The label can help in assessing how dangerous the item is. The word *danger* means that the product is highly toxic, *warning* means that it is moderately toxic, and *caution* means that it is slightly toxic.

- *Avoid aerosol products if possible*, because these disperse their contents in the form of tiny droplets that can be inhaled and subsequently absorbed into the bloodstream.

After purchasing a product, a consumer can help to ensure that it is used safely by following these guidelines:

- *Read the label* to be aware of the product's uses and dangers.

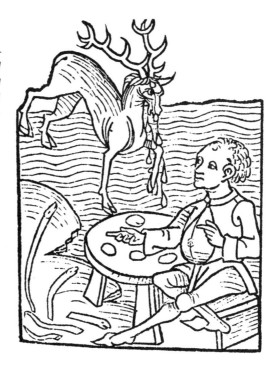

This 15th-century woodcut shows a mythical cure for poisoning: a crystallized tear from a deer bitten by a snake.

- *Follow the label's directions for use* and use only the amount necessary to do the job.

- *Ventilate areas in which poisonous products are used* and work outdoors with the product if possible.

- *Do not eat or drink while using poisonous products* because traces of chemicals can be carried into the eyes or mouth.

- *Clean up after using poisonous products*; this includes making certain that the product has been properly sealed.

Finally, the product should be stored safely to make sure that it does not spill, is not ingested accidentally, and is not used inappropriately.

- *Keep products out of children's reach* by storing them on high shelves or in locked cabinets away from food and drinks.

- *Clearly label all hazardous products* or make sure the original label is on the container.

- *Leave products in their original containers,* and do not remove the label; never put medicines or poisonous products in food or beverage containers.

- *Keep lids and caps tightly sealed* so they will not spill if tipped accidentally and cannot be opened easily by children.

Medicine Cabinet Threat

The bathroom medicine cabinet is the first stop for many people with a minor ache or injury. It can also be the source of a life-threatening emergency, however. Even ordinary drugs, such as aspirin, can be dangerous in a small child's hands. Again, some simple guidelines can help prevent tragedy.

- Make sure that all potentially harmful products have *child-proof closures*—caps that are difficult, if not impossible, for a young child to open.

- *Eliminate* all out-of-date drugs by flushing them down the toilet.

- Give medicine *only to the person for whom it has been prescribed.*

- As with other hazardous substances, keep all medicines in their *original containers* with the *original labels* attached to identify what is inside.

MANAGING POISON VICTIMS

In most instances, poisoning results from negligence or ignorance, and the poison itself is often something purposely kept around the house—often readily at hand.

There are five common ways people are poisoned, whether at home, at work, or elsewhere: ingestion (swallowing the poison), eye exposure, skin exposure, inhalation (breathing the poison in), and intravenous injection (using a needle to take drugs).

The poisoning itself can be either chronic or acute. Chronic poisoning is gradual, occurring through repeated exposure to the substance over an extended period of time. Continued exposure to small amounts of lead in drinking water, for example, can cause brain damage, especially in young children. In contrast, acute effects appear in a severe form in a relatively short amount of time. The poison *cyanide*, for example, can cause death within minutes.

First Aid for Acute Poisoning

In cases of acute poisoning, an onlooker should provide emergency first aid to the victim and summon medical help. When a poison, such as *carbon monoxide* gas, has been inhaled, it is essential to move the victim from the source to prevent further exposure. If the skin is exposed to poison, that area of the body should be thoroughly washed with water, and contaminated clothing should be removed. If the eye is exposed to poison, it should be rinsed with water for 15 minutes.

It is also necessary in poison emergencies to seek trained assistance from the local poison control center. The telephone number for the center should be attached to the phone or placed next to it in a conspicuous location, such as a bulletin board. Every member of the family, as well as baby-sitters, should know where the number is. (These phone numbers are often listed on the inside front cover of the telephone directory white pages.)

When contacting the poison control center, the caller should be ready to give as much information as possible about the emergency, including:

- the name of the poison, including the trade name, if a container listing this information is available
- the ingredients (as listed on the container)
- the amount taken (if known)
- any *antidotes* (substances to counteract the poison) or instructions listed on the container in case of poisoning
- the condition of the poisoning victim, such as whether he or she is conscious or is having convulsions

The caller should also be able to provide the address and telephone number from which he or she is phoning, in case the poison control

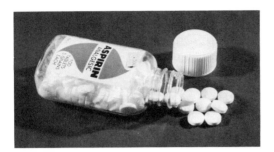

To keep small children from sampling potentially harmful drugs, child-proof caps are installed on medicine bottles.

center must summon help or the line is disconnected and the center needs to call back.

In addition, the medicine cabinet should be stocked with *syrup of ipecac* and *activated charcoal*, poison control products that can be purchased without a prescription at a drugstore. (They should be used under the guidance of a poison control center, doctor, or hospital, since they are not appropriate for all poisoning emergencies.)

Syrup of ipecac, also known as *Brazil root*, is prepared from the dried roots of *Cephaelis ipecacuanha*, a plant found in Brazil and Central America. Ipecac causes vomiting in two ways: by irritating the stomach and by stimulating the vomiting center in the brain. The syrup usually works within 30 minutes, although a second dose may be required.

Ipecac is available without prescription and can be given orally. The oral dose is 2 to 3 teaspoons for children under one year of age and 1 to 2 tablespoons for older children and adults. Vomiting occurs in about 15 to 30 minutes. If the first dose is ineffective, the treatment can be repeated after half an hour. For best results, the person being treated should consume half a glass of lukewarm water after taking ipecac, since vomiting may not occur if the stomach is empty.

As useful as ipecac is, ipecac fluid extract is quite dangerous. This form is 14 times stronger than ipecac itself and may be fatal if consumed, according to *The Pharmacological Basis of Therapeutics.*

Although syrup of ipecac is easy to buy and use, in certain types of poisoning this treatment can do more harm than good. Ipecac should not be used to treat someone who has swallowed a poison that is *caustic*, or burns living tissues. *Acids* and their chemical opposites, *bases*, are both caustic and are often found in cleaning products. Some caustic compounds contain either turpentine (a substance obtained from pine trees) or petroleum solvents (liquids derived from crude oil).

If syrup of ipecac is taken after an individual has swallowed a caustic compound, the vomited material can burn the esophagus, throat, and lips as it returns from the stomach. (If vomiting poses a danger, this information will often be found on a product's label.) The victim should instead be given milk or water to drink—a full pint consumed a quarter of a pint at a time—to dilute the poison.

In addition, vomiting should never be induced in a person who is having convulsions or is not fully conscious, since the individual may inhale the regurgitated material into the lungs.

The other common poison medication, activated charcoal, is a powdery form of carbon produced by heating carbon-based material to high temperatures in the presence of steam and carbon dioxide. The resulting material is extremely porous (containing many internal spaces), which increases the area that is exposed to poisons.

Activated charcoal picks up various drugs and chemicals, allowing these substances to stick to its surface and thereby preventing the body from absorbing them from the intestine. The charcoal can then be safely passed out of the body with the feces. A major advantage of this treatment is that activated charcoal can continue to remove poisons several hours after the charcoal has been swallowed.

The powder, which looks extremely unappetizing, is mixed with water and given to the victim to drink. Children less than five are normally provided with a 30-gram dose in a glass of water; older children and adults normally receive 50 to 100 grams in a glass of water.

Available from local poison control centers, warning labels can help guide children away from the medicine cabinet.

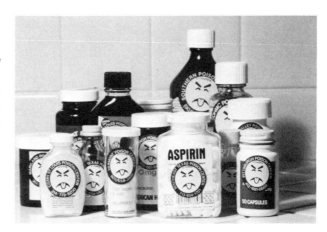

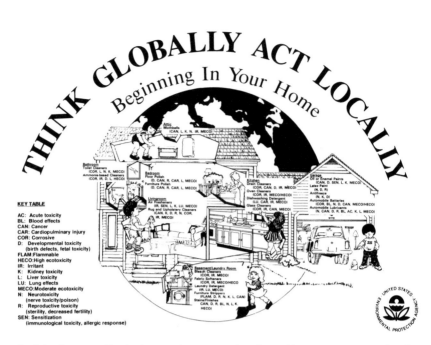

As this diagram illustrates, poisons can be found in numerous parts of the home. Keeping a family safe means knowing where potential dangers exist.

One way to quickly determine the amount of charcoal to add to water is to buy the charcoal in premeasured quantities, such as 25-gram containers, from a pharmacy. Also available is activated charcoal that has already been mixed in liquid. Charcoal should never be used in combination with syrup of ipecac, since the charcoal can pick up the ipecac and reduce its effect.

Along with the above means of poison control, more complex measures must sometimes be used by trained medical personnel to rid the body of dangerous substances. One common method is *gastric lavage*, in which the poison is removed by literally washing out the stomach. A tube is placed down the throat and into the stomach so that the stomach's contents can be siphoned out. Then a cleaning solution is run through the tube and siphoned out again in order to wash out the stomach completely.

Nothing, however, can ensure complete protection from poisons better than knowledge. Educating oneself to the dangers posed by common potential threats is the best insurance against toxic tragedy.

CHAPTER 2

MICROSCOPIC TOXINS

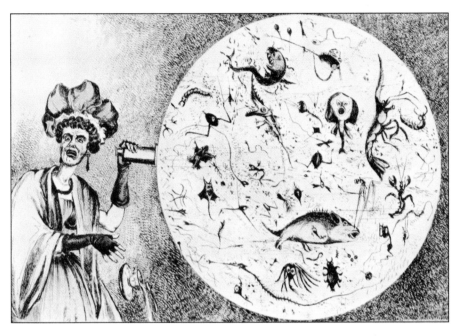

A cartoon from the early 19th century provides a ghoulish satire on the toxic pollution of Britain's Thames River.

Scientists warn that the environment is being poisoned by a lethal buildup of human-generated waste, the by-product of a highly industrialized society. Some of these contaminants take the form of bacteria, which often find their way into the human body as a result of poor sanitation.

TOXINS IN WATER

Unclean water is an efficient transportation system for microbes. Many of the bacteria found in water belong to the family *Enterobacteriaceae* (*entero* means "intestine"), including genera such as *Vibrio*, *Shigella*, *Escherichia*, *Salmonella*, and *Yersinia*. These organisms often inhabit the large intestines of vertebrates and are a source of intestinal disease. In 1990, the federal Centers for Disease Control (CDC) in Atlanta, Georgia, published records showing that from 1986 to 1988 there were 50 reported outbreaks of diseases transmitted by drinking water. These outbreaks caused illness in almost 26,000 individuals.

Dysentery

A bacterium held responsible in four of the outbreaks reported by the CDC was *Shigella sonnei*, an organism that causes a relatively mild form of the disease *dysentery*. Like many disease-causing organisms, it spreads through water contaminated by the feces of infected individuals.

Microscopic view of Shigella *bacteria, various species of which cause dysentery.*

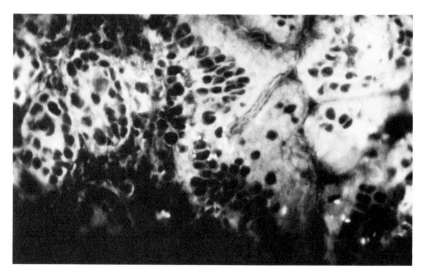

Species of *Shigella* are particularly efficient in causing disease because so few of the organisms are required to start an infection. Although most bacteria need 10,000 to 100 million organisms to initiate an infection, *Shigella* can cause disease in humans with as few as 100 organisms.

Shigella passes harmlessly through the stomach, but once inside the intestines it multiplies and quickly kills the cells lining the intestinal walls. This attack provokes the onset of fever and results in diarrhea containing pus, mucus, and blood.

A related species of bacteria, *S. dysenteriae*, causes a particularly severe form of dysentery. First discovered in 1896 during an epidemic in Japan, the organism produces large quantities of a very dangerous poison called the *Shiga toxin*. Because it kills cells in a specific part of the body (the intestines), Shiga toxin is called a *cytotoxin* (*cyto* means *cell*). Other species of *Shigella* also produce a Shiga-like substance, but they manufacture only about a thousandth as much as *S. dysenteriae*.

In the upper small intestine, Shiga toxin latches onto a *receptor*, a hookup site located on the intestinal cells. Normally, fluid in the small intestine is absorbed into the bloodstream, but the link between the *Shigella* cytotoxin and the intestinal cells interferes with this process. As a result, excess water in the intestines empties out of the body in watery feces, or diarrhea.

The symptoms caused by this disruption of the intestinal cells do not occur suddenly, but only after a 36- to 72-hour delay called an *incubation period*, during which the bacteria establish themselves and multiply. Following this period, the initial symptoms of dysentery appear. Diarrhea causes the victim to lose not only large amounts of water but also essential products called *electrolytes* (substances that take on an electrical charge in solution) dissolved in the intestinal fluid. Because the result, particularly in young or physically weakened patients, can be death, it is important for individuals suffering from dysentery to replace lost nutrients.

Escherichia coli

Escherichia coli, another species of bacteria, wears two faces. The organism is normally harmless and, by making its home in the intestines, protects the digestive tract from colonization by other, harmful microorganisms. *Escherichia coli* first enter a newborn infant through ingested food or water or are passed on to the infant through direct contact with other people.

Certain strains of *E. coli* are not completely benign, however. For example, *enterotoxigenic* forms of *E. coli* (that is, varieties that produce toxins in the intestines) cause diarrhea in infants, as well as in travelers to developing countries who encounter such strains of the organism. These bacteria attach to the intestinal cells by means of tiny hairs called *fimbria* before releasing their toxin.

Cholera

Cholera is caused by the bacterial species named *Vibrio cholerae*, which also spreads most efficiently through contaminated water. This comma-shaped organism, which propels itself with a rapidly moving

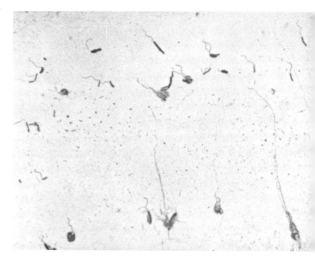

Microscopic photo of Vibrio cholerae. *These bacteria release a cytotoxin that affects cells of the human intestine, causing the disease known as cholera.*

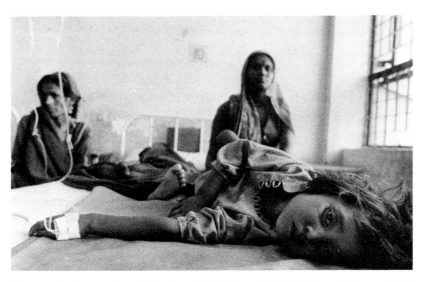

Young cholera patient at a hospital in New Delhi, India, during a 1988 outbreak of the disease.

tail, attaches itself to the cells lining the intestine. Because swallowed water does not remain long in the stomach but passes quickly to the intestine, contaminated water can easily cause infection by *Vibrio cholerae*.

Vibrio cholerae's action is somewhat similar to *Shigella dysenteriae*'s. It too releases a cytotoxin that interferes with the workings of the intestinal cells. As with dysentery, the victim loses large quantities of water and electrolytes. In extreme cases, the organism can cause diarrhea so severe that the victim loses more than 5.3 gallons of fluid per day.

The most recent cholera *pandemic* (worldwide epidemic) began in Indonesia in 1961, swept northward into China, on through Thailand and India, and across to Africa. Within 10 years it invaded Europe, Japan, and the United States. As late as 1983, a small outbreak occurred on an oil rig off the Texas coast. The source was contaminated drinking water, which was then used to cook rice.

TYPHUS

Typhus refers to a group of infectious diseases, including two different forms passed on by the microorganism *Rickettsia prowazekii*. This microbe, which shares characteristics of both bacteria and viruses, is transmitted through the bite of body lice. It is particularly prevalent in crowded, unsanitary areas.

Symptoms of typhus include severe headache; pain in the back and limbs; high fever; a rapid but weak pulse; and trembling in the tongue, which may acquire a whitish coating. In severe typhus, the tongue may turn black and roll up in the back of the mouth. The victim can also experience twitching muscles and become delirious. (In fact, the word *typhus* is taken from a Greek term for "cloudy" or "misty" and refers to the patient's mental condition.) After four or five days, the patient may also develop bluish spots on the body. Complications can affect the lungs and kidneys as well. Although other forms of typhus can be fatal, death occurs mainly in those cases caused by *R. prowazekii*. This bacterium is rarely a source of the disease in the United States, however. Typhus has historically occurred in concentration camps, military installations, nations under wartime occupation, and on crowded ships filled with impoverished immigrants.

TOXIC SHOCK SYNDROME

In 1978, Dr. James Todd, at the Children's Hospital in Denver, Colorado, diagnosed a previously unknown disease in seven children between the ages of 8 and 17. His patients suffered from high fevers—above 102°F (39°C)—nausea, vomiting, diarrhea, extreme lethargy (drowsiness), a rash followed by skin peeling, and a sudden drop in blood pressure. In severe cases the drop in pressure caused *shock*, which means that an inadequate blood supply deprived the heart, brain, and other organs of oxygen and nutrients. If left untreated, shock can rapidly lead to death. The illness was named *toxic shock syndrome* (TSS).

Dr. Todd suspected the bacterium *Staphylococcus aureus* as the cause of TSS, and subsequent studies confirmed that suspicion. By the end of 1980, doctors in the United States had identified a total of 941 cases of TSS. By 1990, more than 2,500 cases had been diagnosed. In about 95% of the cases, the victims were women, and 90% of the cases occurred in menstruating women who were using tampons, particularly those made with a new, superabsorbent material.

Because tampons block the elimination of blood from the vagina, they can provide a breeding ground for bacteria. It is believed that *S. aureus* that breed under these conditions pass through the vaginal wall and into the bloodstream, where they produce a toxin that causes blood vessels to leak. This apparently results in reduced blood pressure and, in turn, shock.

Crowded, unsanitary areas, such as this Manhattan neighborhood in the 1880s, are good breeding grounds for disease-causing microorganisms.

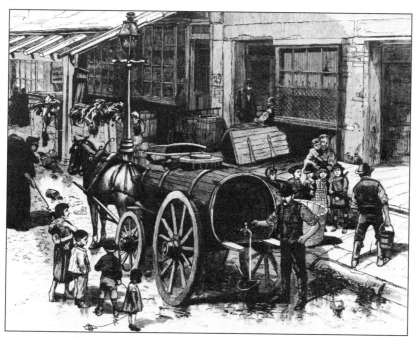

The elimination of superabsorbent tampons from the market, and more careful use of tampons in general by women, has decreased the incidence of TSS associated with menstruation. In addition, women who regularly use tampons are learning to rely on them for only part of the menstrual cycle and to change them frequently. However, the rate of TSS in men and nonmenstruating women has not decreased, so that these individuals now account for more than 20% of TSS cases. Fortunately, about 99% of adults are immune to the disease.

TSS has occurred after staphylococcal infections of cuts, burns, and surgical incisions. It has also been associated with the use of vaginal contraceptive sponges. A particularly intriguing form of TSS occurs when persons already suffering from influenza become infected with *respiratory* (lung) staphylococci. Some experts have suggested that this sort of "double" infection was the cause of a devastating plague that occurred in Athens in 430 B.C. This postinfluenzal TSS has been named the *Thucydides syndrome*, after the ancient historian who recorded the event.

CHAPTER 3

CONTAMINATED FOOD

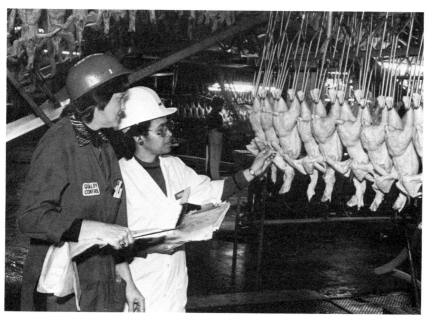

Careful inspection of food-processing plants is an important defense against dangerous microorganisms in the food supply.

To meet the nutritional needs of growing populations, industrialized nations have developed complex processing and transportation systems to get raw food from the farm to store shelves. These methods usually work efficiently to provide fresh produce and properly preserved food. But errors in the process can lead to contamination of food by *pathogenic* (disease-producing) microorganisms, which are widespread in the environment, in animals, and in humans.

Food contaminated by pathogenic microbes often causes illness because of the toxins released by these organisms. Consuming these organisms or the toxins they produce commonly results in diarrhea, vomiting, or both. Some forms of food contamination affect parts of the body aside from the digestive tract, such as the nervous system.

Estimates of the number of cases of *food-borne gastroenteritis* (inflammation of the stomach and intestinal lining due to illness carried by food) occurring in the United States vary widely, from 6.3 million to 81 million cases each year, according to a report in the medical journal *The Lancet* (September 29, 1990). The huge difference in numbers reflects the various methods of estimation and calculation used. The estimated number of deaths from food-borne illness also varies, according to *The Lancet* report, from 523 to 7,041 per year.

In addition to causing human suffering, food-borne illnesses are costly in terms of such factors as medical care, lost work, and payment of damages to people who have become ill after using a manufacturer's food product. Again estimates vary, ranging from $7.7 billion to $23 billion per year.

SALMONELLOSIS

Among the most common and costly of food-borne diseases is *salmonellosis*, a form of gastroenteritis caused by bacteria belonging to the genus *Salmonella*. These rod-shaped microbes contaminate poultry, egg products, raw milk, and meat.

The estimated annual cost of salmonellosis in the United States is about $1.4 billion, or approximately $700 per case. A survey conducted by the U.S. Centers for Disease Control of food-borne disease cases occurring between 1983 and 1987 found that *Salmonella* accounted for 57% of the bacterial disease outbreaks for that period. It was the most frequently reported bacterial pathogen for each of those years. According to the U.S. Food and Drug Administration (FDA), it is estimated that 2 million cases of salmonellosis occur annually in the United States.

Development of salmonellosis requires the ingestion of anywhere from one million to one billion *Salmonella* organisms. Many of the

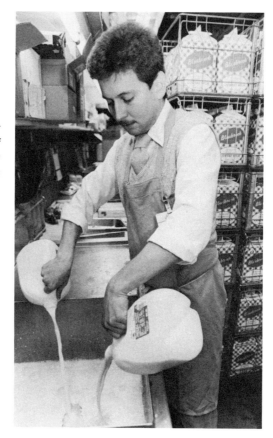

A food store manager dumps quantities of suspect milk during a 1985 salmonellosis outbreak in Illinois.

bacteria do not survive the acidic conditions of the stomach. Those that do, however, undergo an incubation period—during which they reproduce in the intestine—lasting from 8 to 48 hours. Following this, the bacteria penetrate the cells lining the end of the small intestine and the beginning of the large intestine.

After invading the intestinal cells, the bacteria trigger a response from the body's immune system. This, in turn, causes fluid to be secreted into the intestine. The result is diarrhea, which usually lasts from three to four days, and seldom longer than a week.

In 1985, medical laboratories confirmed 16,659 cases of salmonellosis traced to improperly pasteurized milk in Illinois (although it has been estimated that as many as 197,581 people were actually affected).

The contamination occurred in a state-of-the-art milk processing plant in Illinois that served hundreds of dairy farms. The processing equipment included 400 miles of stainless steel pipes, 638 valves, a giant holding tank, and more than 600 large metal plates. Despite the technology, a malfunction of valves permitted raw milk contaminated with *Salmonella* to enter a pipeline carrying pasteurized milk.

Contaminated Meat

Bacteria of the genus *Campylobacter* are another common source of gastroenteritis in the United States. Indeed, researchers have found *Campylobacter* contamination in up to 90% of some stocks of chicken and turkey ready to be shipped to market.

Poultry meat can be contaminated during the rapid, mechanical procedure of killing, plucking, and slicing the chicken, when feces containing the bacteria can get on the meat. Other types of meat have also become tainted during butchering or packing. Machinery contaminated by cattle or mice feces, scraps, and blood adds to the spread of bacteria.

A condemned side of beef; organisms such as Campylobacter *and* Salmonella *can attack meat, poultry, and other foods.*

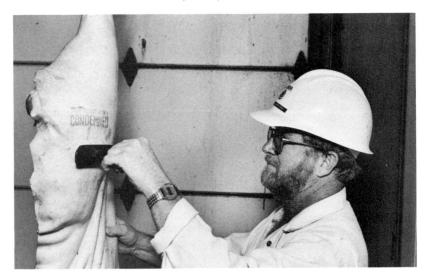

FOOD INTOXICATION

Efforts to preserve food and prevent spoilage stretch back to prehistory, when primitive people preserved food that was harvested or slaughtered by such methods as drying and cold storage in dark caves. A more elegant method of preservation was developed during the late 18th century by a sweets manufacturer from France named Nicolas-François Appert (ca. 1750–1841). His discovery involved preserving food in bottles, a technique that came to be known as *canning*. By 1824 he had perfected the process well enough to preserve about 50 different types of foods. His methods benefitted the French dictator Napoleon Bonaparte, who had been having great difficulty providing his armies with edible provisions and who realized the need to preserve food for long periods of time.

The canning process involves heating food to kill contaminating microorganisms. This system is usually successful, but when it goes awry, either through negligence or an equipment breakdown, unwary consumers can suffer a very distressing, and in severe cases fatal, bout of food poisoning.

Clostridium Botulinum

A major threat in improperly canned food is the bacterium *Clostridium botulinum*, an organism that is *anaerobic*, meaning that it can live without oxygen. As a result of this characteristic, these bacteria can survive inside sealed food cans. If the cans are improperly processed, the bacteria thrive and produce a deadly nerve toxin that causes *botulism*. Because it is the toxin that causes the disease, and not the bacteria themselves, botulism is referred to as a form of *food intoxication* rather than food poisoning.

Symptoms of botulism, which usually appear about a day after *C. botulinum* is ingested, include weakness, dizziness, constipation, and severe dryness of the mouth. Blurred vision then develops, along with general muscle weakness, speech difficulties, and an inability to swallow. The condition eventually leads to *respiratory paralysis*, a failure of the muscles that control breathing.

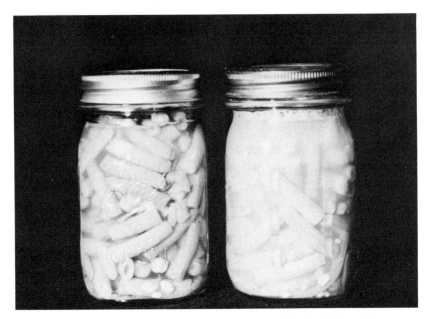

The cloudy appearance of a liquid that normally should be clear—as in the bottle on the right—is a sign that the product may be contaminated with Clostridium botulinum, *the bacterium that causes botulism. The organism, which can survive without oxygen, is a major threat in canned food.*

A characteristic of the botulism toxin is that it is *heat labile*, meaning that it is destroyed at high temperatures. However, heat treatments of canned foods must be carried out properly to inactivate the toxin, which can survive heat that kills the botulism bacteria themselves. Boiling home-canned vegetables or processed fish for 10 minutes just before consuming them destroys the toxin. Food prepared in factories or at home should be heated for 20 minutes at 79°C or for 5 minutes at 85°C in order to inactivate the toxin.

The *C. botulinum* toxin is among the most powerful biological toxins known to science. A single microgram (one-millionth of a gram) is nearly enough to kill a human. Indeed, American troops stationed in Saudi Arabia during the 1991 conflict with Iraq were supplied with vaccines against this toxin as a safety measure in case of biological warfare.

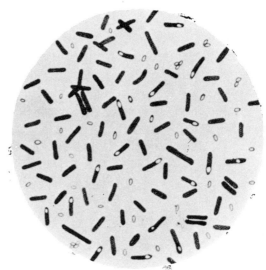

Microscopic photo of Clostridium botulinum.

In contrast to its presence as a contaminant in canned or bottled food, *C. botulinum* is normally present in natural food sources. The organism is widely distributed in soil, lake bottoms, and on vegetation, and is therefore occasionally found in the intestines of mammals, birds, and fish. Originally, uncooked meat or sausage (the Latin word for sausage is *botulus*) were among the most common sources of botulism. Since 1950, most cases of the disease have been caused by foods prepared at home or in small catering units rather than in those that have been commercially processed.

CIGUATERA: TOXIN FROM THE SEA

Ciguatera poisoning is the most frequently reported food-borne disease associated with seafood consumption in the United States. The fish involved tend to be large, bottom-dwelling creatures, such as barracuda, red snapper, amberjack, and grouper. Indeed, because barracuda are so frequently contaminated, Miami has banned their sale. During the 1970s there were 94 outbreaks of ciguatera poisoning, totalling 418 cases, recorded by the U.S. Centers for Disease Control. Most of the cases were diagnosed in southeastern Florida and in Hawaii.

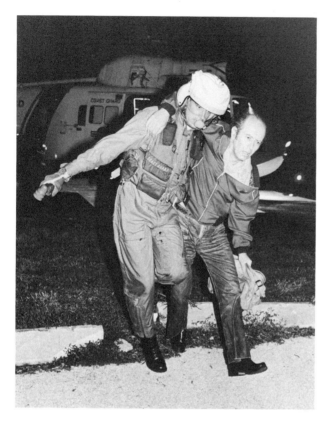

A coast guardsman in Miami helps a crew member from an Italian supertanker. In 1982, this crewman and four others were flown from the tanker to Miami for medical care after they and others on the ship became sick from eating contaminated barracuda.

The culprit in this seafood-borne disease is *ciguatoxin*, a poison that is not only unaffected by heating, freezing, or storage but can survive for weeks. In addition, it does not alter the taste, color, or odor of contaminated fish. Ciguatoxin is produced by tiny plantlike organisms called *dinoflagellates*, especially members of the species *Gambierdiscus toxicus*. Herbivorous (plant-eating) fish that eat these dinoflagellates absorb the toxin and, when the fish in turn are eaten, pass it on to larger, carnivorous (meat-eating) fish.

Although the fish themselves are not affected by the poison, humans who eat the tainted fish develop nausea, vomiting, abdominal cramps, and diarrhea within about six hours. Later, muscle pain, weakness, sweating, and chills may occur. Major *neurological* (nervous-system-related) symptoms include itching and unusual sensations around the mouth, hands, and feet. For example, hot and cold sensations may be reversed: patients often perceive cold drinks to be hot and carbonated in their mouth.

Victims may also have the illusion that their teeth are loose and may feel a burning sensation in their feet. Joint pains, blurred vision, sensitivity to light, and temporary blindness are other common symptoms of ciguatera poisoning. In particularly severe cases, the toxin causes a decrease in heart rate and blood pressure, eventually paralyzing respiratory function. Symptoms usually disappear within eight days, and deaths are rare.

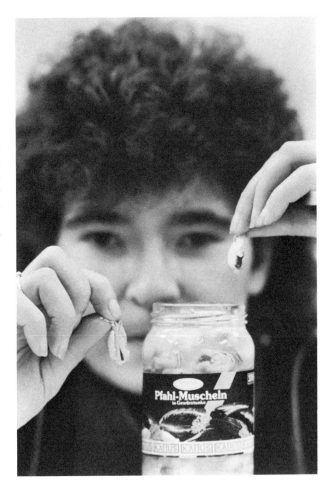

In 1987, bottled mussels from Spain were removed from store shelves in Germany after the shellfish were found to be contaminated with a deadly neurotoxin.

SHELLFISH

Mussels, clams, oysters, and scallops—all seafood mainstays—can prove to be a health hazard if they have been contaminated by certain free-floating dinoflagellates. This is especially true of such shellfish that have been tainted by the species of dinoflagellate known as *Gonyaulax catenella*, which is abundant in latitudes above 30 degrees north (above Florida) and below 30 degrees south (the southern tip of Africa). When dinoflagellates bloom in large numbers on North American beaches, they often cause the so-called red tides. (Not all red tides are contaminated by poisonous organisms, however.)

Signs of food poisoning begin within a half hour of eating contaminated shellfish. These symptoms include *paresthesia* (abnormal sensations, such as burning or tingling) involving the head, hands, and feet, frequently accompanied by nausea, vomiting, and diarrhea. In extreme cases of shellfish poisoning, muscle paralysis develops and leads to difficulty or pain in speaking, swallowing, and breathing. If the episode is particularly severe, breathing difficulty causes death within 12 hours.

CHAPTER 4

ANIMAL TOXINS

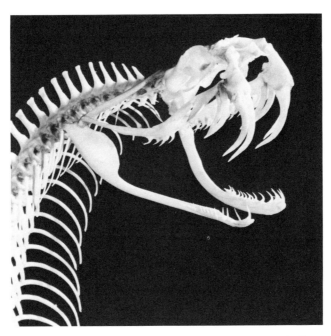

There are about 20 species of venomous snakes in the United States. These reptiles inject poison into their victims through venom glands connected to long, curved fangs.

Animals have evolved a variety of means both to protect themselves and to catch food. These include fast flight, strong bodies, sharp claws and teeth, and, in many cases, chemicals that poison an animal's adversaries or its prey. A toxin secreted by an animal and passed to a victim through a bite or a sting is called a *venom*.

VENOMOUS SNAKES

In the United States today, there are about 20 species of venomous snakes—that is, snakes that use their fangs to inject venom into the body of their adversaries and prey. Each year in the United States, venomous snakebites cause about 15 fatalities, according to the book *Snakes of the World*, by Christopher Mattison. In India, where venomous snakes are more abundant and many people live in rural areas, it is estimated that about 10,000 to 12,000 deaths from snakebite occur annually.

The evolution of poisonous snakes may initially have been related not to protection but to digestion. Because snakes tend to swallow their quarry whole, they need powerful digestive *enzymes* (proteins that induce chemical reactions in the body without themselves being changed) to break down food. It has been suggested that, by chance, some of the enzymes that developed were also strong poisons that could leave the snake's prey weak or unable to move. A further advantage developed when the long, curved teeth that some venomous snakes used to grab hold of their victims evolved into needlelike fangs. These fangs developed channels through which the poisonous venom could travel as the snake bit into the flesh of its victim.

The salivary glands of venomous snakes also evolved, becoming larger and developing a separate area where venom could be stored until needed. (When a rattlesnake strikes, for example, its fangs sink into its prey and its muscles contract, squeezing a venom gland in each cheek. The poison is forced through the narrow tube that runs from the gland to the fang.) Furthermore, these sharp fangs could move forward, allowing the snake to strike with a stabbing motion. These developments also gave the snakes in which they occurred a newfound defense mechanism against enemies.

The substances that can make up the venom of a particular type of snake include a bewildering array of chemicals. Tissue-destroying enzymes found in snake venom include *hyaluronidase*, *protease*, and *phospholipase*. The exact combination of enzymes varies from snake to snake, but generalizations can be based on the two basic groups of

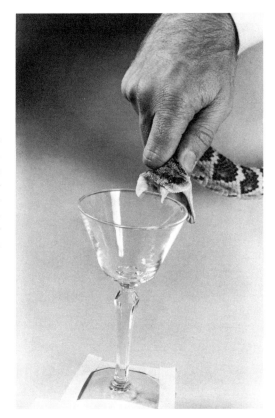

Venom being "milked" from a rattlesnake; snake venom contains powerful enzymes that appear to have initially evolved to help these reptiles digest their prey, which had to be devoured whole.

venomous snakes: the *Crotalidae* (pit vipers) and the *Elapidae* (coral snakes and Asian cobras).

Pit vipers include rattlesnakes, water moccasins, copperheads, and pygmy rattlesnakes. This family derives its name from the deep pits, each containing a heat-sensitive organ that is located between its members' eyes and nostrils. (These organs help the pit vipers hunt warm-blooded prey.) Pit vipers range over the entire United States, except for Alaska, Maine, and Hawaii. In general, the venom of these snakes consists mainly of *hemotoxic* poisons, which act principally in the circulatory system, destroying red blood cells and capillary walls. (Capillaries are small blood vessels that connect arteries with veins.) Such venom can cause internal bleeding, a drastic decrease in blood pressure, and shock. Other toxins in the venom cause nausea, vomiting, and fainting.

Coral snakes, which are confined to the Americas, inhabit the southern and southwestern United States and are found in countries as far south as Argentina. True coral snakes inject a venom that is *neurotoxic*, acting mainly on the nervous system. Its effects include numbness, weakness, poor muscle coordination, difficulty in swallowing and speaking, visual disturbances, breathing problems, and convulsions. In 1990, there were 18 reported coral snake bites in the United States, according to the American Association of Poison Control Centers.

Cobras also have dangerous neurotoxic venom. These snakes, known for their neck ribs, which can expand to form a hood of skin, are found in warm regions of Africa and Asia. Cobra bites are fatal in at least 10% of victims. The king cobra, found from southern China to the Philippines and Indonesia, is the world's largest venomous snake, often reaching a length of more than 12 feet. The spitting cobra of southern Africa has fangs that are pointed forward. It can project its venom accurately at its victim's eyes from distances of more than seven feet.

SNAKEBITES: HOW DANGEROUS?

It may be surprising to know that in many cases of snakebite, potentially deadly snakes appear to release little or no poison during an attack. Perhaps, at least in some instances, the snake is saving its

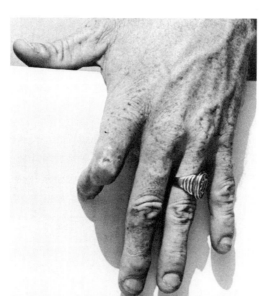

A rattlesnake's venomous attack destroyed tissue and bone in this man's index finger, leaving the digit withered and inflexible. A poisonous snake does not, however, necessarily release venom with each attack.

venom for the animals it intends to use as food. (This is not to suggest that someone who is bitten by a snake should not seek immediate medical help, since the effects of such attacks are unpredictable.)

In their book *Venomous Reptiles*, coauthors Sherman A. Minton, Jr., and Madge Rutherford Minton illustrate how greatly the effects of snakebite can vary. They recount the story of three people who were bitten by the same rattlesnake within a period of about 15 seconds. The first person apparently suffered no symptoms at all, but the second and third did, although one of them had a complete recovery within 24 hours.

Treating Snakebites

Before being given first aid, a person who has been bitten by a snake should be moved out of danger of a second bite and should then be transported as quickly as possible to a physician. When the snakebite is serious, the major treatment is *antivenin*, a mixture of *antibodies* (natural disease-fighting agents) that counteract the venom. If it will not delay the patient's trip to the hospital, or if the patient cannot immediately reach a doctor, it may be helpful to apply a tourniquet (a device that restricts the flow of blood, such as a broad band of fabric) on the injured limb above the bite area. This will deter poison from traveling through the bloodstream to the heart and then being pumped to the rest of the body. However, the tourniquet must be loosened at intervals, perhaps every 10 minutes, to prevent gangrene (tissue decay caused by obstruction of the blood supply). The recommendation of removing snake venom by making an incision (cut) at the site of a bite and applying suction has become less popular, partly because it can increase the risk of infection.

SPIDERS

The dry, dimly lit corners and crevices of houses, barns, and woodpiles are potential homes for a variety of unwanted pests that crawl, hop, and spin webs. Perhaps as much as snakes, venomous spiders have captured the popular imagination. Although most spiders do carry some sort of venom, only a few species are truly dangerous.

The venom glands of the spider are typically somewhat cylindrical and covered by muscle. Each gland is connected by a duct to a separate fang. Spiders appear to be able to voluntarily contract the muscles covering their venom glands, which means that, like snakes, these insects seem capable of controlling whether or not they inject venom into a victim during an attack and how much venom will be secreted.

The Black Widow

Throughout the United States, especially in southern states, the female black widow spider, or *Latrodectus mactans*, quietly spins her web and awaits a male suitor. After mating, the female often kills and devours her partner, leaving her a "widow."

Immediately recognizable by her shiny black body with a red hourglass-shaped marking on the abdomen, the female black widow

Black widow spiders; the larger specimen is the female, and the smaller is the male. The bite of the female releases a neurotoxin that can cause severe symptoms in humans.

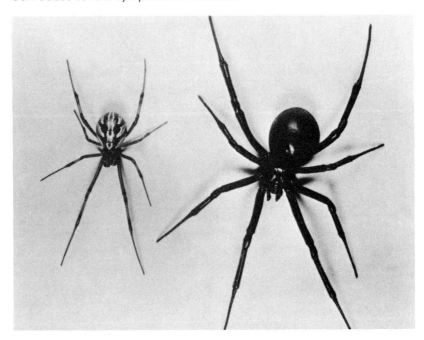

spider releases a *neurotoxin* that causes severe symptoms in humans. Following an attack by this spider, the victim feels a slight pain where bitten. The pain then rapidly progresses to the chest, abdomen, and joints. Nausea follows swiftly, along with a tendency to salivate and sweat. Breathing, or *respiration*, becomes difficult, and the muscles of the abdomen, chest, or back become rigid. The bite is rarely fatal, however, and recovery is usually complete within a week. When death does occur, the victims are primarily very young children, the elderly, and people with high blood pressure. According to the 1990 study, by the American Association of Poison Control Centers, more than 2,400 black widow bites, but no fatalities, were reported in 1990.

The Brown Recluse

The bite of the brown recluse spider, or *Loxosceles reclusa*, also brings dramatic and painful symptoms. Like the black widow's bite, an attack by this spider, which is found in the south-central United States, is rarely fatal, and most deaths occur in small children.

The brown recluse's venom produces a reddened area around the bite, which evolves into a blister. Within two days of the bite, symptoms such as fever, chills, weakness, nausea, vomiting, and joint pains may develop. These often disappear by themselves, but some physicians advocate treating the victim with drugs known as *steroids* to relieve these effects or surgically removing the bitten area. Almost 1,400 brown recluse bites, but no related deaths, were reported in 1990, according to the AAPCC.

SCORPIONS

Scorpions are another venomous resident of the southern United States, including Arizona, New Mexico, and California. They carry a neuro-toxin, dispatched from a stinger at the end of a curved tail. A scorpion attack can cause intense pain followed by numbness, drowsiness, restlessness (in children), lockjaw (in which the jaw muscles go into continuous and extreme contraction), extremely high fever, and bleed-

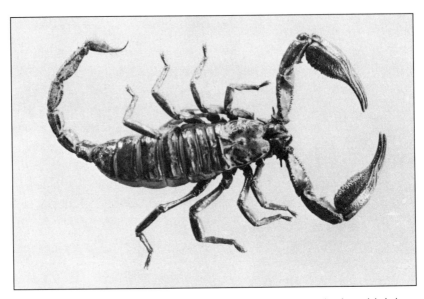

Like black widow spiders, scorpions also carry a neurotoxin, which is dispatched from a stinger at the end of their curved tail.

ing into the lungs and intestines. In severe cases, the victim may have convulsions. More than 5,800 scorpion stings, but no deaths, were reported in 1990, according to the AAPCC.

VENOMOUS AND TOXIC MARINE ANIMALS

There are roughly 1,000 species of marine animals known to carry venom or to be somehow poisonous, according to *Marine Toxins and Venomous and Poisonous Marine Animals*, by Findlay E. Russell. The AAPCC study indicates that more than 1,900 exposures to marine animal poisons were reported in 1990, although no deaths resulted in any of these cases.

Studying marine venoms is particularly difficult, according to Russell, because the chemical composition of these poisons can vary not just from one species of marine animal to the next but also between members of the same species. This can make it hard for scientists to understand precisely how marine venom acts on an animal's prey. Moreover, the higher up the evolutionary ladder the creature is, the more complex its venom tends to be.

The severity of the effects of a toxin also vary a great deal from one marine animal to the next. The venom of some water-dwelling creatures merely causes blood vessels to temporarily dilate (widen) or constrict (narrow), whereas the venom of other such creatures can have more serious effects on either the circulatory or nervous system.

Jellyfish

In 1978, a five-year-old boy was frolicking waist deep in the waters off an Australian beach when he was stricken by the darts of a jellyfish. The boy ran from the water screaming in pain and tugging at translucent tentacles stuck to his legs. The young victim, whose legs and abdomen were covered with large red welts, received emergency care at a hospital within 20 minutes of the accident. Despite heroic efforts by the doctors to administer drugs, oxygen, and electric shocks to revive the boy's heart, he died of heart failure.

The youngster was a victim of *Chironex fleckeri*, commonly called the box jellyfish or sea wasp. This species delivers powerful stings by means of thousands of tiny darts, called *nematocysts*, located on its tentacles. The darts release a *cardiotoxin*, a poison that causes the circulatory system to fail. Usually, the symptoms of a jellyfish sting begin immediately and include stinging, burning, and sometimes severe pain, along with an itchy rash.

In the warm waters off the east and west coasts of Australia, at least one or two bathers fall victim to *C. fleckeri* stings each summer. Many others are injured but survive. A closely related species, *Chiropsalmus quadrigatus*, found in the Philippines, is also deadly. (The jellyfishlike Portuguese man-of-war, genus *Physalia*, is another deadly creature. In the United States, this blue-colored creature is found along the shores of Florida and other southern and Gulf Coast states.)

Jellyfish belong to the phylum Cnidaria, so-called because the small, poisonous stingers, or nematocysts, that its members possess are also called *cnidae*. In addition to causing heart failure, cnidae venom can cause muscle spasms (sudden, painful muscle contractions) and *anaphylaxis* (an immediate and often lethal allergic reaction to a poison caused by a previous exposure to that substance). The severity of a jellyfish sting depends on the species involved, the number of stingers discharged into the skin, and the sensitivity of the victim to a particular venom.

Puffer

Most cases of food poisoning are accidental, but in Japan the *puffer*—a fish that contains a deadly neurotoxin (tetrodotoxin) far stronger than cyanide—is a delicacy. The most poisonous parts of the animal include the liver, ovaries, and intestines, although toxicity varies among the approximately 100 species of this fish. The *Fugu rubripes*, or *tiger fugu*, is especially coveted among diners. (*Fugu* is the Japanese term for "puffer.")

In Japan, a puffer meal, often served in thin, raw slices, is prepared by trained chefs skilled in finding the nontoxic portions of the fish. Despite the care taken in preparing puffer, the process is not foolproof. According to an article in *Business Week* magazine (May 28, 1990), a "handful" of Japanese die each year from eating the fish. Most of these people, however, are fishermen who fail to prepare their catch properly.

The meat of the puffer fish is considered a delicacy, but if improperly prepared, it can prove deadly because of a toxin 500 times stronger than cyanide.

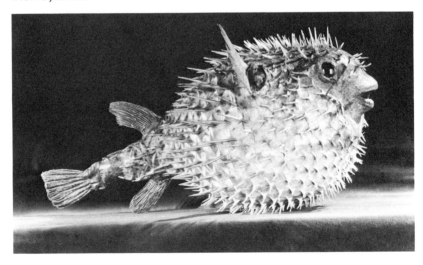

CHAPTER 5

POISONOUS PLANTS

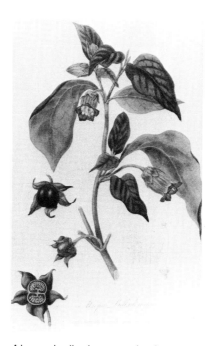

Atropa belladonna, *also known as deadly nightshade, contains the toxin atropine throughout all of its parts.*

Because increasing numbers of Americans have come to live in cities and suburbs, away from heavily wooded areas, the danger of plant poisoning is not as great as it once was. Yet the 1990 study by the American Association of Poison Control Centers indicates that more than 100,000 plant-related poisonings were reported in 1990 (although only three deaths were recorded).

EVOLUTION OF PLANT POISONS

Plant toxins probably evolved with the adaptation of plants to life on land after their initial evolution in water. The various chemical, or *metabolic*, reactions that occur in plant cells produce toxic by-products. Aquatic plants can eliminate these poisons in water, but terrestrial plants are forced to hold on to their toxins. To prevent these harmful substances from causing damage, plants either evolved ways to turn poisons into nontoxic compounds or began to store them in some part of the plant, such as the bark, where they would pose no danger to the rest of the plant. This last strategy had a second advantage: it provided a defense against plant-eating insects. Some of the poisons that developed in this way were also harmful to larger animals, including humans.

THE SOLANACEAE FAMILY

Several members of the plant family, known as Solanaceae (which includes the potatoes) have long histories as "magic" plants used by witches and sorcerers. Among these are henbane (*Hyoscyamus niger*), belladonna (*Atropa belladonna*), and mandrake (*Mandragora officinarum*). Their reputation arises from the high concentrations of *hallucinogens*—compounds that produce hallucinations—they contain.

Atropa belladonna, also known as deadly nightshade, contains, throughout all of its parts, a toxin called *atropine*. Atropine produces its major effects by blocking the function of certain *neurotransmitters*, chemical substances that carry messages from one nerve to another. By interfering with these chemicals, atropine paralyzes the part of the nervous system called the *parasympathetic nervous system* (which controls some of the body's involuntary functions). The principal effects of atropine poisoning are delirium, fast pulse, and fever.

Despite the danger posed by this toxin, modern doctors have put some of its effects on the parasympathetic nervous system to productive use. Because atropine dilates the *pupil* of the eye (the opening in the *iris*, or colored part, of the eye), ophthalmologists use it to aid examination of the *retina* (a section of the eye behind the pupil, where the image formed by the eye's lens is projected). Atropine also relieves symptoms of hay fever and head colds by drying up nasal and tear duct secretions. Atropine can also be used to treat bowel spasms caused by overactivity of the parasympathetic nervous system.

STRYCHNOS NUX-VOMICA

The poison *strychnine* occurs in the seeds of the *Strychnos nux-vomica* tree, native to India. The word *vomica*, which means "depression" or "cavity," refers to an indentation in the seed that according to legend marks the imprint of God's finger.

Although strychnine has no demonstrated medical use, this poison is now employed as a garden and agricultural pesticide to kill rats and

The poisonous mushroom Amanita muscaria. *Even experts have difficulty identifying which mushrooms are poisonous and which are safe to eat.*

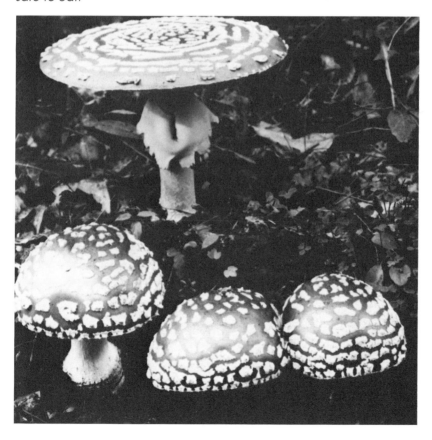

other ground animals. Even this limited use occasionally leads to accidental poisoning of children.

The gastrointestinal tract rapidly absorbs strychnine, which then enters the bloodstream. From there, the poison is quickly absorbed by the body. Strychnine's action on the *central nervous system* (the brain and spinal cord) causes nerves to become particularly excitable, throwing the body into spasms and convulsions.

The first symptoms of strychnine poisoning occur within a half hour and include agitation and apprehension, followed by pain and stiffness in the muscles of the face and mouth and in the muscles around the backbone. Next, spasms of the muscles that control respiration begin to cause *cyanosis* (a bluish tint to the skin caused by too little oxygen in the blood) and *apnea* (an absence of breathing). In addition, the victim typically suffers a series of as many as 10 convulsions, interrupted by periods of muscle relaxation and extreme exhaustion lasting about 10 minutes, during which time the person experiences extreme pain.

Most victims of strychnine poisoning survive this series of seizures, which can last as long as six hours. A long seizure may, however, cause death from apnea. In the case of a massive overdose of strychnine, apnea occurs within minutes of ingestion. Apparently, this is because nerves in the *medulla*—the portion of the brain that controls breathing (among other functions)—are affected. Although only 26 cases of strychnine poisoning were cited in the AAPCC study, 4 of them resulted in death.

MUSHROOMS CAN KILL

In the summer of 1990, a French book publisher suspended sales of the newest edition of its dictionary because the pictures of several mushrooms had been mislabeled. More than an embarrassing error, the mistake was potentially deadly: the book identified some of the most poisonous mushrooms on earth as safe to eat.

Mushrooms are classified as a type of *fungus*, which means that they are plantlike, but are not classified as true plants. Of the more than 30,000 species of large mushrooms, however, only a few are dangerous. But the threat of poisonous mushrooms (some of which are commonly called toadstools) has been aggravated in recent decades by people's growing enthusiasm for organic foods as well as experimentation with mushrooms containing natural hallucinogens. Even expert *mycologists*, scientists who study fungi, have difficulty identifying which mushrooms are poisonous. Thus, an amateur mushroom gatherer cannot be sure that each specimen in his or her collection of wild mushrooms is safe to eat. Mushrooms accounted for 9,570 reported plant-related poisonings in the AAPCC study, but only one death.

Mushroom poisoning is especially prevalent during the fall, when the large reproductive part of the fungus, the caplike top, can be easily harvested. Unfortunately, the most poisonous species of mushroom closely resemble some of the most popular edible species. There are no simple rules of thumb to help the amateur avoid poisonous mushrooms, except the dire folk warning:

> There are old mushroom hunters,
> And there are bold mushroom hunters,
> But there are no old, bold mushroom hunters.

By far the most common culprits in mushroom poisoning are species belonging to the genus *Amanita*, such as *Amanita phalloides*,

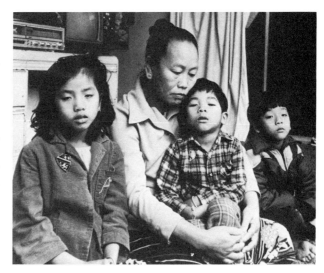

Following an incident of accidental poisoning in 1983, a woman waits with her three grandchildren to learn more about her daughter, who was hospitalized after eating toxic mushrooms at a party.

known as the destroying angel or deathcap mushroom. The poison produced by *A. phalloides* harms its victims by damaging the membranes and nuclei of cells.

The symptoms of anatoxin poisoning appear within 24 hours of eating the mushroom and include abdominal pain, severe vomiting, diarrhea, and fever. By the third or fourth day, liver and kidney failure occur, followed by coma and death. Ingestion of only a single mushroom cap containing anatoxin may prove lethal.

Other species of *Amanita*, such as the fly mushroom (*Amanita muscaria*) and panther mushroom (*Amanita pantherina*), contain substances known as *muscarinic toxins*, which are neurotoxins. These cause tearing of the eyes, excessive salivation, nausea, headache, blurred vision, vomiting, abdominal pain, bronchospasm (a rapid, repetitive contraction and relaxation of muscles of the air passages leading to the lungs), slowing of the heart rate, and shock. Most muscarinic toxins produce symptoms within minutes or hours.

WELL-KNOWN BUT DEADLY PLANTS

What do Christmas and the Greek philosopher Socrates (c. 470–399 B.C.) have in common? Each is closely linked to a potentially deadly plant.

Long considered to be a romantic symbol of Christmas, *mistletoe* was known for centuries before the birth of Jesus and by 1597 had made its way into herbal encyclopedias. In his book *The Herball, or generall historie of plantes*, the English botanist John Gerard (1545–1612) warned his readers of the dangers of eating mistletoe. He stated that the plant "inwardly taken is mortall, and bringeth most greevous accidents, the toong [tongue] is inflamed and swolne [swollen], the mind is distraughted, the strength of the hart and wits faile."

In addition to this dreadful description of the popular holiday shrub, the North American mistletoe, *Phoradendron serotinum*, also bears the reputation of being a parasite of evergreen trees and shrubs. Common from New Jersey and southern Indiana southward to Florida and Texas, this species contains toxic chemicals in all parts of the plant, especially the berries. Other species occur throughout the continent.

Poisonings from mistletoe have occurred when people eat the berries or drink a tea made from the fruit. The symptoms of mistletoe poisoning include intestinal pain, diarrhea, and a slow pulse. In addition, the victim may suffer nausea, vomiting, difficult breathing, and even delirium. In extreme cases, mistletoe poisoning can be fatal.

Hemlock

Another toxic plant known to ancient civilizations is *hemlock*, or *Conium maculatum*. It is also called poison fool's parsley because it is a member of the same family as the herb parsley. Originally a native of Eurasia, *C. maculatum* provided the poison that killed Socrates. The authorities, alarmed by his radical teachings, decided to put an end to his influence by sentencing him to death. As was the custom, Socrates performed his own execution by drinking a poisonous concoction made from hemlock.

The Death of Socrates, *by Jacques-Louis David (1748–1825). The Greek philosopher, sentenced to death for his radical teachings, committed suicide by drinking a concoction made from the toxic plant hemlock.*

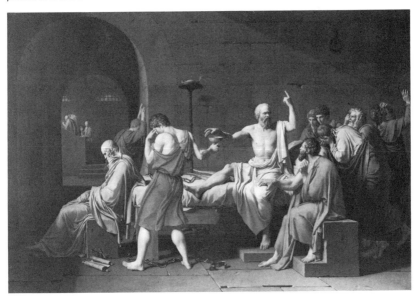

Conium maculatum has large leaves, white flowers, and hairless, purple-spotted or -lined hollow stems that can grow several feet tall. The water hemlock, or *Cicuta maculata*, which looks similar to its cousin fool's parsley, is also toxic. These plants should not be confused with the nonpoisonous evergreen trees called hemlock, which grow in North America and Asia.

The toxin in hemlock plants is called *coniine*. This poison paralyzes peripheral muscles, such as those in the arms, hands, and legs. Other common symptoms of hemlock poisoning are abdominal pain, nausea, vomiting, and fever. Eventually, muscle paralysis causes fatal respiratory failure (in which the individual cannot breathe properly or at all).

Coniine was the first *alkaloid* to be synthesized in the laboratory. (Alkaloids are substances found in plants and used in a variety of pharmaceuticals; they include caffeine, nicotine, and morphine.) This synthesis, accomplished in 1886, was a major step in the study of alkaloids and their properties.

CHAPTER 6

POISONOUS METALS

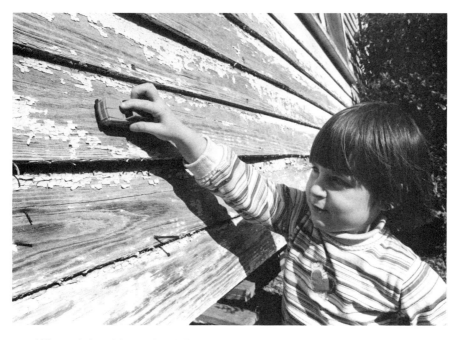

Although lead-based paints are now banned, some can still be found on the walls of older homes. This presents a particular danger to young children, who may chew chipped wall paint.

When Lewis Carroll's storybook heroine Alice attended a Wonderland tea party, she was perplexed by the behavior of the Mad Hatter. This strange man was excitable, irritable, and perhaps even suffered from hallucinations. Eccentric as he was, however, his behavior was grounded in reality.

The reality was that hatmakers in the 19th century sometimes used a special mercury compound to treat the beaver fur used in making hats. Because mercury, like many metals, is potentially poisonous, mercury fumes that some of these workers inhaled led to symptoms similar to those of the Mad Hatter. This chapter will examine several of the more widespread metals that cause toxic reactions.

MERCURY

A tragic example of mercury poisoning occurred four decades ago in Minamata Bay, Japan. During an eight-year period starting in 1953, more than 40 people died of exposure to the toxic metal, and almost 70 individuals—mostly children—were left handicapped. The problem became known as *Minamata disease*. Eventually, an estimated 1,000 deaths or more in the Minamata Bay area were blamed on mercury poisoning.

The poison was carried in fish eaten by the victims or their pregnant mothers. The outbreak of the disease was traced to a factory that had released mercury waste into the bay.

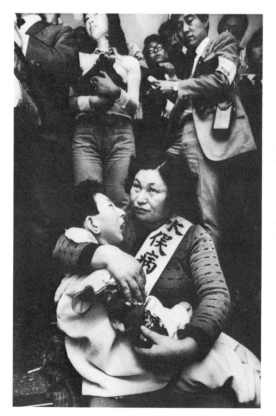

This photo, of a mother holding her severely handicapped daughter, demonstrates the tragic consequences of mercury poisoning in Minamata Bay, Japan, during the 1950s.

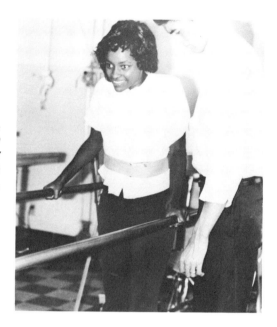

In this 1970 news photo, a New Mexico woman works toward recovery after falling victim to mercury poisoning.

Mercury is widely used to manufacture chemicals, paints, pesticides, and *fungicides* (chemicals that kill fungi, such as molds). In those industries that utilize mercury, workers can suffer chronic poisoning by breathing in vapor or dust containing the metal. Poisoning has also occurred among persons who have eaten grains treated with mercury fungicides. More than 2,200 cases of mercury poisoning were reported in 1990, according to the American Association of Poison Control Centers. Two deaths resulted.

Ingestion of mercury causes the sudden onset of severe symptoms, including abdominal pain, vomiting, and bloody diarrhea. In addition, the metal damages the kidney, thus causing a serious reduction in the output of urine. In such cases, death can occur from *uremia*, an excess of waste products in the blood.

Depending on the form of mercury to which an individual is exposed, the metal may remain in the body for many weeks. This is because mercury can bind itself to fats and proteins in cells and eventually reach a high concentration in the liver and brain. Nerve cells, particularly those in the brain, are especially vulnerable to mercury damage. As a result, physical coordination, vision, and hearing can all be affected. Mental function may also suffer, leaving the victim anxious, irritable, and forgetful.

ALUMINUM

Crude aluminum, first isolated from the naturally occurring substance aluminum oxide in 1825 by Danish physicist Hans Christian Ørsted (1777–1851), has become one of the most commonly used metals in the United States. Although pure aluminum is weak and soft, this silvery white metal becomes hard and strong when it is mixed with small amounts of other metals in the fused materials known as *alloys*. Aluminum is used in airplane parts, building materials, refrigerators, air conditioners, cooking utensils, and many other products.

Despite its numerous benefits, aluminum may lead to several sorts of health problems. Because it dissolves in acid, cooking acidic foods

At one time, aluminum poisoning could occur through hemodialysis, because the metal was found in the fluid and equipment used in the process. Copper poisoning was another problem in hemodialysis, because copper tubing was once part of the equipment. Both substances have since been removed from dialysis instruments.

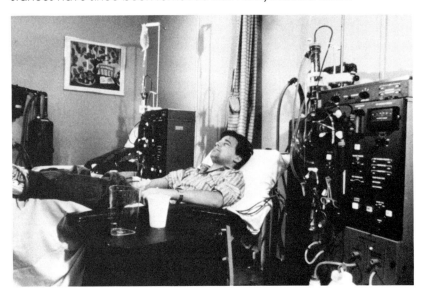

such as tomatoes in aluminum pots and pans can lead to ingestion of this metal in the diet. Consumed in large quantities, aluminum can irritate the digestive system. Ironically, certain antacid tablets contain *aluminum hydroxide* to neutralize digestive acids in the stomach. Some experts suggest that these antacids be avoided.

Aluminum has also been found in fluid used for *hemodialysis*, a technique for cleansing waste products from the blood of persons whose failed kidneys can no longer perform this function naturally. Moreover, some dialysis patients take aluminum salts to help rid their body of excess phosphorus, which builds up when their kidneys fail. For certain hemodialysis patients, however, exposure to aluminum can result in *anemia*—an abnormally low number of red blood cells—because the metal apparently interferes with chemical substances in the body that stimulate red blood cell production. It can also cause *dialysis dementia*, a form of brain damage similar to that found in *Alzheimer's disease*, a progressive brain disease that robs victims of their intellectual abilities. (Today, aluminum-free dialysis fluid is available, and alternative medication is available to reduce phosphorus in the body.)

In fact, aluminum may play a role in Alzheimer's disease. Researchers have found concentrations of the metal in damaged brain areas of persons who have the disease.

ARSENIC

The ancient Greeks and Romans used the metal arsenic as both a healing agent and a poison. The history and folklore surrounding arsenic prompted *pharmacologists*—scientists who examine how drugs work—to undertake intensive studies of this substance. Through such research, chemist Paul Ehrlich (1854–1915) pioneered the study of *chemotherapy*, the use of chemicals as medicines. In 1909, Ehrlich also developed the first successful treatment for the sexually transmitted disease *syphilis*, which consisted of an arsenic-containing drug called arsphenamine.

Today, *arsenicals*, medicines that use arsenic to achieve their effects, are employed only in the treatment of certain tropical diseases. Arsenic can also be manipulated to form a gaseous substance called *arsine* that has been used as a military poison. In addition, arsenic is used in insecticides, weed killers, paint, wallpaper, ceramics, and glass. It also is released into the environment as a by-product of *smelting*, in which the rocky ores of various metals are heated to release pure copper, lead, zinc, and other metals.

Poisoning occurs when arsenic interrupts the chemical reactions that release energy from food. Once ingested, arsenic can become concentrated in areas such as the hair and fingernails. It may remain in the hair for years. Arsenic is also deposited in bones and teeth. Among those persons who may be exposed to this poisonous metal are agricultural workers coming into contact with insecticides that contain arsenic.

The sudden ingestion of a large dose of arsenic causes violent gastroenteritis, vomiting, and diarrhea, followed by convulsions. Eventually, the victim lapses into a coma and, if not adequately treated, can suffer heart failure resulting in death. Ingestion or inhalation of smaller quantities of arsenic over a longer period of time causes nervous system symptoms such as burning pains in the hands and feet. According to the AAPCC study, 504 cases of arsenic poisoning (not including individuals who were poisoned by pesticides containing arsenic) were reported in 1990, resulting in 7 deaths.

LEAD

The hazards of lead poisoning have been known for at least 2,000 years. The Greek physician Dioscorides (c. 40–c. 90) noted both mental and physical deterioration in patients who ingested lead or inhaled lead fumes. The Romans used lead in building the aqueducts that carried water to their cities and to produce eating utensils and wine cups. Some historians attribute the fall of the Roman Empire in part to a feeblemindedness of the ruling class caused by lead poisoning.

Today lead is still used in a variety of products, including batteries, ammunition, protective shielding for nuclear power plants, leaded glass, some types of gasoline, insecticides, and coverings for electrical cables. Lead soldering is found in a small percentage of food cans, and lead is contained in the glazing that covers some domestic and imported

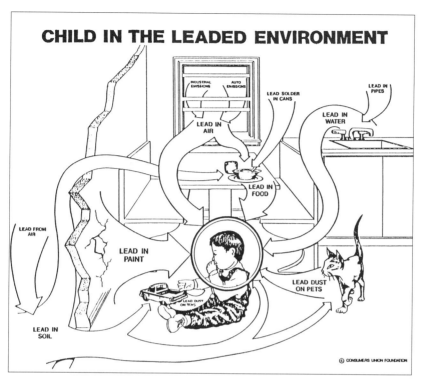

CHILD IN THE LEADED ENVIRONMENT

As this diagram indicates, lead in the environment can find its way into the human body through a number of different sources.

pottery (although in 1991 the U.S. Food and Drug Administration limited the amount of lead allowable in ceramic glazing.) Not surprisingly, people still suffer lead poisoning by breathing auto exhaust fumes that contain the metal or by consuming lead-contaminated food. One way in which lead can work its way into the food chain is through animals that feed on plants and pasture grass exposed to lead fumes.

The metal also appears in tap water, leaching out of lead pipes and the lead solder used on brass fixtures in homes. As a result, the federal government has directed water suppliers to reduce lead concentrations to 15 parts of lead per 1 billion parts of water by the year 2014, or to replace the water pipes. Some lawmakers, environmental groups, and public health experts have criticized the proposal because the rules will not have an impact for a number of years. They also point out that state health departments will be required to take on a heavy financial burden to oversee the new federal regulations.

A particularly tragic problem is the lead poisoning of young children who chew on chips of wall paint in old houses. Before 1945, most types of paint were made with lead. Although the federal government declared lead-based paint a health hazard 20 years ago, hundreds of thousands of homes still contain it. As late as 1991, the secretary of Health and Human Services called lead poisoning "the number one environmental hazard facing our children." In California, a study conducted between 1987 and 1990 found evidence that more than half a million one- to six-year-old children in that state may be in danger of neurological and behavioral difficulties as a result of lead poisoning.

Lead has far-reaching effects on the body because it hinders the regulatory system that keeps cells healthy. It also interferes with the

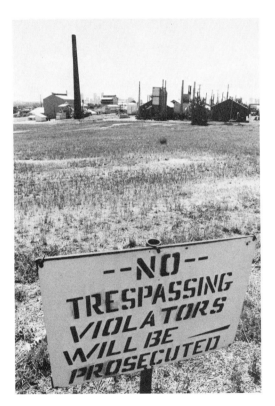

The danger of metallic contamination of the environment is clear in this photograph warning persons away from a smelter plant that has released high concentrations of vanadium, cadmium, arsenic, lead, and zinc into the surrounding area.

action of enzymes in the body. Symptoms of lead poisoning include abdominal pain, a metallic taste in the mouth, vomiting, diarrhea, black feces, and coma. In addition, exposure to substantial quantities of lead in air, food, dust, and drinking water can delay mental and physical development in babies, impair mental abilities in children, and cause anemia, kidney damage, and hearing loss in children and adults.

Early symptoms of chronic lead poisoning, which can occur in industries where workers inhale lead fumes over a long period of time, include loss of appetite, weight loss, constipation, irritability or apathy, fatigue, headache, and anemia. In its advanced stage, chronic lead poisoning can paralyze leg and arm muscles. Severe poisoning can impair the ability to walk and see and may cause convulsions. Chronic lead poisoning can also disturb kidney function. More than 2,000 cases of lead poisoning were reported in 1990, according to the AAPCC, but no deaths were recorded.

In the late 1970s, while living in California, Don and Fran Wallace began suffering from a baffling deterioration in health. Don's own detective work at last turned up the cause: lead poisoning. The couple, who by then had moved to Seattle, traced the source to a set of terra-cotta dishes they had been using. The glazing on the dishware contained lead.

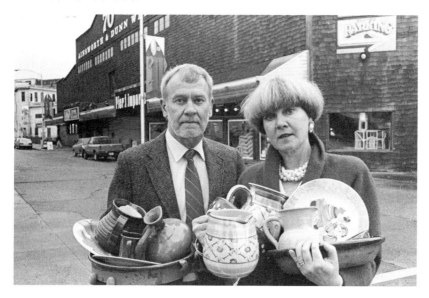

COPPER

A common source of metal poisoning is the use of copper-containing food cans, jar lids, and cooking utensils. If allowed to sit for a long enough time, acidic foods or beverages can, for example, leach copper out of copper-containing pots. Moreover, as with aluminum, dialysis was formerly a source of copper poisoning because of the copper tubing used in the process. Today, however, dialysis tubing no longer contains this metal.

Acute copper poisoning causes headache, dizziness, a metallic taste in the mouth, excessive salivation, stomachache, nausea, vomiting, diarrhea, and general weakness. As the disease progresses, the heart may begin to race, and the blood pressure can soar. Damage to the liver and kidneys, organs where copper tends to accumulate, may also occur. If the symptoms of copper poisoning are mild within six hours of their first occurrence, the patient is likely to recover. In cases of severe poisoning, however, death may occur within a week.

Major consequences can also result from *Wilson's disease*, an inherited disorder that prevents the liver from effectively ridding the body of excess copper and in turn allows the metal to build up in the liver and brain. During childhood, Wilson's disease victims suffer severe liver damage. In older children and young adults, the disease causes various problems related to the nervous system, such as tremors, difficulty in walking, talking, and eating, and *chorea* (unpredictable, rapid, and jerky movements). According to the AAPCC there were 771 copper poisonings reported in 1990, but no deaths.

CHAPTER 7

POISONOUS COMPOUNDS AND GASES

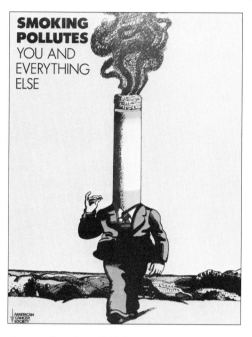

SMOKING POLLUTES YOU AND EVERYTHING ELSE

According to a 1989 government report, tobacco smoke contains more than 40 carcinogenic chemicals.

Although the harmful effects of some substances have been known for many years, the toxic consequences of others have been discovered only recently. In the latter case, the poison, such as asbestos or lead, may have been widely used by industry for years, requiring a costly cleanup.

TOBACCO SMOKE

Cigarette smoking is thought to be responsible for more than one out of every six deaths in the United States. Smoking and other types of tobacco use are implicated in four of the leading causes of death in the United States: heart disease, cancer, stroke, and chronic obstructive lung diseases (such as chronic bronchitis and emphysema).

According to a 1989 report by the U.S. Surgeon General, tobacco smoke contains more than 40 chemicals considered to be *carcinogenic* (cancer-causing). It also contains:

- nicotine, a drug occurring naturally in tobacco leaves, which stimulates the nervous system

- tiny particles of *tar,* a waste product of burning tobacco, which fill the alveoli (air holes) in the lungs, interfering with respiration

- carbon monoxide gas, which is also produced by burning tobacco (and will be further discussed in the section below) and decreases the amount of oxygen the bloodstream can carry. This in turn affects the functioning of the heart, leading in some cases to heart attack.

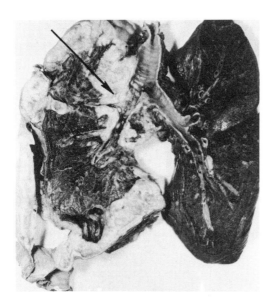

Lung cancer in a heavy smoker. Smoking and other types of tobacco use are also implicated in such common killers as heart disease, stroke, and chronic obstructive lung disease. Arrow indicates location of cancer.

In addition to its effects on smokers, tobacco can also harm developing fetuses. Research indicates that the newborn infants of women who smoke cigarettes tend to weigh less than the infants of nonsmokers, a problem that appears to be related to a reduced supply of oxygen reaching the fetus. Additionally, the babies of cigarette smokers have an increased chance of suffering from brain and psychological disorders and of exhibiting lower intelligence. Beyond this, smoking during pregnancy has been linked to *sudden infant death syndrome*, in which a baby dies suddenly and without explanation.

CARBON MONOXIDE

Carbon monoxide (CO) gas is colorless, tasteless, and odorless. Since it is also toxic, it can be present in dangerous concentrations without an individual's being aware that he or she is being exposed to it. As CO floods the lungs and passes into the bloodstream, it can suffocate its victim. This occurs because CO attaches to *hemoglobin*, the substance in red blood cells that normally carries oxygen from the lungs to the tissues, thereby preventing the hemoglobin from performing this life-sustaining function.

Carbon monoxide is given off naturally by a variety of sources. For example, it is produced both by forest fires and by microorganisms that live in the ocean. But humans are responsible for about 10% of the CO found in the atmosphere, because the gas is produced when substances such as coal, oil, gasoline, or wood are burned. Another significant— but avoidable—source of CO is cigarette smoke.

At a level of 0.05% CO in the air, a person doing light work for one hour may suffer a slight shortness of breath and a minor headache. Longer exposure to CO causes nausea, irritability, chest pain, confusion, and greater difficulty in breathing. Another common symptom at this stage of CO intoxication is cyanosis, a bluish tinting of the skin caused by a shortage of oxygen. When CO concentrations rise beyond 0.1%, the symptoms of intoxication intensify dramatically, leading to unconsciousness and ultimately to death.

In the case of chronic CO poisoning, in which an individual is repeatedly exposed to small concentrations of carbon monoxide over a long period, the toxin gradually damages the nervous system, affecting memory and causing general mental deterioration.

According to the AAPCC, more than 7,500 cases of carbon monoxide poisoning were reported in 1990, including 26 fatalities.

RADON

Radon 222 is a toxic, radioactive gas that, like carbon monoxide, is tasteless, colorless, and odorless. It is given off by uranium 238, which occurs naturally and quite commonly in rocks and soil. Because uranium is so prevalent in the environment, radon gas is found in buildings throughout the United States, creeping in through basement drains and cracks and infiltrating underground wells. Radon testing has revealed harmful levels of this substance in many schools, and research indicates that dangerous levels may occur in at least 1 in 10 American homes.

When radon is inhaled, it decays in the lungs, releasing radiation that can harm lung tissue. Eventually, such exposure can result in lung cancer. The U.S. Environmental Protection Agency estimates that radon gas is responsible for 20,000 lung cancer deaths annually.

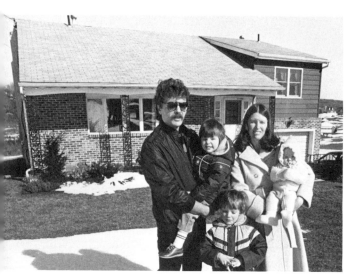

This home in Boyertown, Pennsylvania, was one of the first American homes found to be contaminated with toxic radon gas. Prevalent in the environment, radon can creep into homes through basement drains and cracks and can infiltrate underground wells.

If a house is found to be contaminated with radon, the problem can often be alleviated by proper ventilation, which will prevent the gas from accumulating indoors. If radon has been found in well water, special filters can be used to remove it from the water.

CYANIDE

In 1988, the Middle Eastern nations of Iran and Iraq were at war. In a battle over disputed territory, chemical weapons were dropped on the Iraqi town of Halabja, about 10 miles from the Iranian border. Among the toxic substances used, apparently, was *hydrogen cyanide* (HCN), or *prussic acid*. (To this day there is a dispute over whether Iran or Iraq was responsible for the chemical bombardment. The number of dead is also in question, with estimates ranging from hundreds to thousands of civilians.)

Along with its grimmer uses, cyanide also has practical applications. Thus, hydrogen cyanide gas is used for fumigation (disinfecting or destroying pests). Cyanide also plays a role in the production of synthetic rubber, fertilizer, and various chemicals. In addition, it is used for cleaning metal and in the process of refining gold and recovering it from ore.

Moreover, cyanide occurs naturally in certain foods. For example, some varieties of lima beans, especially those that are native to the Caribbean, contain harmful levels of cyanide. Soaking and cooking the beans, however, removes much of the poison. By contrast, the varieties of lima bean grown in the United States contain only negligible quantities of cyanide, and federal law prohibits anyone from marketing beans that contain harmful concentrations of this substance.

Besides its presence in some types of lima bean, the seeds of apples, cherries, peaches, apricots, and plums contain substances that release cyanide during digestion, but these seeds are only dangerous if their coverings, or capsules, are broken.

Acute cyanide poisoning, the result of either inhaling or ingesting the substance, immediately causes the victim to lose consciousness. Convulsions occur, and the poison may prove fatal within 1 to 15 minutes. In smaller doses, the effects of cyanide can be slower, with the victim suffering dizziness, flushing, headache, drowsiness, rapid respiration, vomiting, a drop in blood pressure, and, finally, unconsciousness. In most cases of fatal cyanide poisoning, convulsive death occurs within four hours. If the victim survives beyond this time, recovery usually follows. There were 442 cyanide poisonings reported in 1990, according to the AAPCC, including 14 deaths related to the substance.

ASBESTOS

Known since ancient times for its resistance to fire, the mineral *asbestos* gets its name from the Greek word meaning "inextinguishable". Although it was valued by ancient peoples—such as the Romans, who used asbestos to make tablecloths that could be cleaned by fire—it did not become a major industrial raw material until the early 20th century.

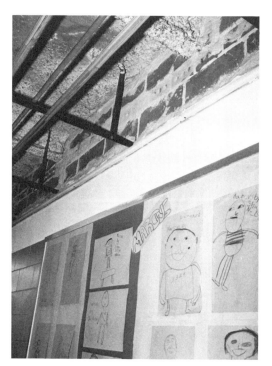

A 1978 news photo of asbestos insulation in the ceiling of a New York public school. Inspections required under the federal government's Asbestos Hazard Emergency Response Act found crumbled asbestos in 45,000 of the nation's schools.

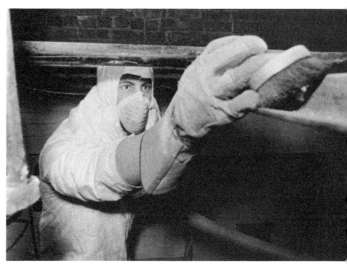

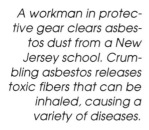
A workman in protective gear clears asbestos dust from a New Jersey school. Crumbling asbestos releases toxic fibers that can be inhaled, causing a variety of diseases.

Eventually, however, asbestos came to be found almost everywhere: in clothing, cement, home and school insulation, brake linings, and plumbing insulation. This widespread use of asbestos has created a number of potential perils. As early as 1907, medical reports described scarring in the lungs of asbestos workers. In 1935, asbestos was associated with cancer of the bronchi (air passages leading to the lungs), and in the 1960s, comprehensive studies of the general population clearly showed that asbestos fibers pose a danger to the general population. Particularly notable findings during this decade were reported by Dr. Irving Selikoff and his colleagues at the Mount Sinai Medical School in New York City. These researchers supported the theory of a *dose-response model*, which suggests that the bigger the dose of asbestos, the more likely a person is to get an asbestos-related disease.

Selikoff's group found that asbestos textile weavers, pipe insulators, and shipyard workers suffered unusually high rates of cancer, especially in the lining of the lung or abdominal cavity. This type of cancer, called *mesothelioma* and virtually unknown before the 20th century, can occur after prolonged exposure to even low levels of asbestos. If the disease grows unchecked, it can crush the lungs.

The mechanism by which asbestos causes mesothelioma and lung cancer is not yet known. Moreover, the long lag time between exposure to asbestos and the onset of disease has often delayed public recognition of the health threat posed by this popular building material. Yet by the 1980s, mesothelioma was thought to be killing between 1,000 and 3,000 people in the United States each year. (Death estimates vary because the disease is difficult to diagnose.) Among asbestos workers—especially industrial workers who smoke—lung cancer is even more common than mesothelioma.

Another asbestos-caused disease, called *asbestosis*, or *pulmonary fibrosis*, produces scarring of the lungs among people who have had a relatively high degree of exposure to asbestos over a period of 15 to 40 years. (The disease rarely occurs in anyone who has not worked with asbestos or with products containing the material.) The primary symptom of asbestosis is *dyspnea*, or difficulty in breathing. Other symptoms include clubbed fingers and a reduction in the amount of air the lungs can hold. As with mesothelioma, the odds of getting pulmonary fibrosis from exposure to asbestos are greater in persons who smoke. In one study, nonsmokers who had been exposed to asbestos for 20 years did not have pulmonary fibrosis, but 29 out of 45 smokers who were exposed for the same length of time did have the disease.

Asbestos poisoning can affect those who have mined the mineral, worked with it in industry, or have been exposed to its fibers in other ways, such as from flaking ceiling tiles. In the 1980s, both the U.S. Occupational Safety and Health Administration and the Environmental Protection Agency became increasingly involved in efforts to protect people from asbestos exposure. In 1986, Congress passed the Asbestos Hazard Emergency Response Act (AHERA), which required inspections of schools for asbestos. If asbestos material is found to be a hazard in a school, it must be removed.

Simply having asbestos in a building is not necessarily dangerous, however. The problem occurs if an asbestos-containing material has become *friable*—that is, if it will crumble easily, releasing asbestos fibers that can be inhaled. A 1984 report from the Environmental Protection Agency indicated that more than 730,000 public and commercial buildings in the United States (not counting schools) had friable asbestos-containing materials.

Some scientists have argued that leaving asbestos in place in some schools is safer than the risk of dispersing its fibers into the air during its removal. Another debate centers on whether all types of asbestos cause mesothelioma. Certain studies indicate that some forms of asbestos are less efficient in causing the disease, even at high concentrations. Yet many public health experts believe that all varieties of asbestos found in schools are capable of causing mesothelioma.

POLYCHLORINATED BIPHENYLS

Polychlorinated biphenyls (*PCBs*) are a family of more than 200 different toxic, oily compounds containing chlorine, hydrogen, and

In this 1986 news photo, a Detroit resident watches as a government-hired cleanup firm fences her property off from an alley contaminated with PCBs. In this instance, the toxic compound, which can cause liver damage, apparently came from a scrap metal yard.

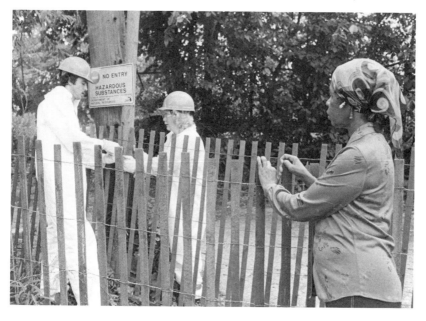

carbon, with the carbon atoms arranged in ringlike structures called phenyls, from which the names of these compounds are derived.

Because PCBs can withstand high temperatures without breaking down into other substances, they were useful for many applications. They were employed in insulation for electrical equipment as well as in paints, adhesive material, caulking compounds, and other products. By the 1960s, scientists realized that PCBs were toxic and remained in the environment for a long time. By then, however, tens of millions of pounds of these materials had already been produced, much of which had been released into the air, earth, and water. Although PCB production ended in 1977 and importation of PCBs into the United States was banned in 1979, the long life and 40-year history of use of these compounds suggest that they will continue to pollute the environment for many years to come. Sources of PCB pollution have included sewage vents, industrial and municipal disposal systems, leakage from dumps, and burning refuse.

Since 1967, scientists have found PCBs in a variety of foods. Their journey through the food chain can, for example, begin when PCBs in water are consumed by microscopic organisms that are, in turn, eaten by fish that end up in the human diet. In addition, PCB-containing paint in feed silos has contaminated grain stored in the silos, tainting the milk and eggs produced by farm animals that have consumed the grain. Not surprisingly, PCBs have also turned up in human tissue and in the milk of nursing mothers. One 1977 study found PCBs in polar bears at the top of the Arctic food chain.

Prolonged exposure to PCBs causes skin irritation and severe liver damage as well as swelling of the kidneys and heart. Exposure to PCB vapors plugs glands in the skin, causing the skin to erupt with pinhead-to pea-sized *cysts* (abnormal, fluid-containing sacs). The cysts eventually grow into larger, pus-filled sacs. Meanwhile, the liver damage caused by PCBs leads to drowsiness, indigestion, nausea, and *jaundice*—a yellowing of the skin caused by accumulation of the pigment *bilirubin* in the bloodstream. Ordinarily, the blood transports bilirubin to the liver, where it is broken down chemically and excreted in a digestive substance called *bile*.

About half of all patients who have been treated for liver damage linked to PCBs or related compounds have died, according to the *Handbook of Poisoning: Prevention, Diagnosis, & Treatment.* Yet people who work with such chemicals are likely to recover if they are removed from exposure as soon as they develop skin cysts. Nevertheless, the fact that PCBs persist in unchanged form in human fat for years has made many scientists concerned that they may lead to cancer or—because PCBs can be passed from a pregnant woman to her fetus—cause mutations in offspring.

PCB-related illnesses occurred in Japan in 1968 and Taiwan in 1979, according to the publication *Scientific American Medicine* (published by Scientific American, Inc.). These outbreaks were traced to cooking oils contaminated with PCBs and related chemicals. Taiwanese children who were exposed to the poison before birth suffered from a number of problems, including abnormally low birth weights and inflammation around the eyes. Later, these children tended to have high rates of bronchitis, and 10% showed various nervous system problems, such as slowed development of coordination and speech, as well as impaired intelligence.

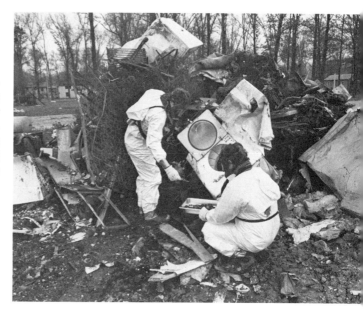

In 1983, federal technicians took soil samples to determine whether flooding in dioxin-contaminated Times Beach, Missouri, had caused the toxic chemical to spread.

DIOXIN

A dramatic illustration of a toxic chemical's far-reaching effects can be found in the story of Times Beach, Missouri. In 1982 and early 1983, the federal government evacuated all 2,240 residents of the town from their homes forever. The culprit in this environmental tragedy was *dioxin*, a chemical compound—known technically as 2,3,7,8-tetra-chlorodibenzo-para-dioxin—that has no use. It exists only as a contaminant produced during the manufacture of pesticides and other products. During the 1970s, however, a waste hauler sprayed dioxin-tainted oil on the streets of Times Beach in order to control dust. In 1991, plans were completed for tearing down the town's buildings and burning the contaminated soil of Times Beach.

Dioxin continues to cast a chilling shadow. During the Vietnam War, the compound Agent Orange was used as a *defoliant*, a substance

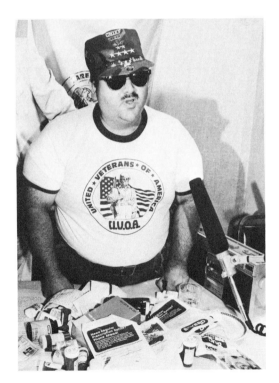

At a 1984 press conference in Washington, D.C., a Vietnam War veteran displayed medications that, he said, were required by his physical condition. According to the veteran, his health was impaired by exposure to Agent Orange during the war.

that removes leaves from trees, by the U.S. military. Sprayed in Vietnam over a period of eight years, Agent Orange defoliated trees that provided cover for enemy soldiers. Only later was it discovered that dioxin was a by-product of the manufacture of Agent Orange. Dioxin went on to become the center of a battle between the federal government and Vietnam veterans claiming to suffer from exposure to Agent Orange. The debate about whether dioxin has caused increased cancer rates among Vietnam veterans continues to this day.

Studies do show that dioxin is the most powerful cancer-causing chemical ever tested in laboratory rodents. However, reports have differed about whether and to what extent dioxin causes cancer and other serious diseases in humans. In 1991, the *New England Journal of Medicine* reported on the largest study ever performed of dioxin exposure in the workplace. The research involved 5,172 male workers at 12 plants that produced chemicals contaminated with dioxin.

According to the study, cancer deaths among workers who had been exposed to dioxin were about 15% higher than expected. The higher death rate occurred mostly among men exposed to dioxin for more than a year and in whose blood the quantity of dioxin was probably as much as 500 times higher than in the general population. For these particular workers, the cancer death rate was 46% higher than expected.

Though the study reported in the *New England Journal of Medicine* does not prove that dioxin causes cancer in humans, it does support the theory. There is a growing consensus that dioxin is in fact dangerous to humans and that long periods of continued exposure to it, or short periods of high exposure, are probably responsible for increased rates of cancer. Moreover, research suggests that dioxin can depress the body's immune system.

DEADLY SOLVENTS

In 1861, the German chemist Friedrich August Kekule von Stradonitz (1829–96) fell asleep in front of a fireplace and had a vision of a flame, in the shape of a snake, joining its ends to form a ring. Awakening from his nap, von Stradonitz knew he had the answer to a problem that had long puzzled him. He had been trying to figure out the shape of the molecule of *benzene*—a substance that was known to contain six carbon atoms and six hydrogen atoms. Von Stradonitz's dream told him that benzene existed as a ring.

Today, benzene and two similar chemicals, *toluene* and *xylene*, are commonly used in industry. These compounds, which are liquid at room temperature, are used as solvents, or substances in which other materials can be dissolved. They are especially useful in the production of plastic cement and rubber, and in fact toluene is the ingredient abused by glue sniffers attempting to get "high."

Inhaling large amounts of benzene, toluene, or xylene can depress the activity of the central nervous system and cause brain damage, resulting in *ataxia*, or loss of coordination of movement. Mild exposure to these chemicals causes dizziness, weakness, euphoria, nausea, and vomiting. There is a tightening of the chest and staggering during walking.

Greater exposure causes more severe symptoms, which include blurred vision, shaking, and difficulty in breathing. Eventually the heart beats irregularly, and the victim suffers paralysis and convulsions before lapsing into unconsciousness. Persons who inhale even small amounts of benzene, toluene, or xylene over a long period of time can turn pale and suffer headache, loss of appetite, drowsiness, and nervousness. Prolonged exposure can also lead to anemia and affect the ability of the bone marrow to manufacture blood cells.

In addition to these effects, benzene, toluene, and xylene also cause skin irritation on contact, leading to scaling and cracking of the skin, and benzene is a known carcinogen, having been found to cause leukemia in humans.

CHAPTER 8

DRUG POISONING

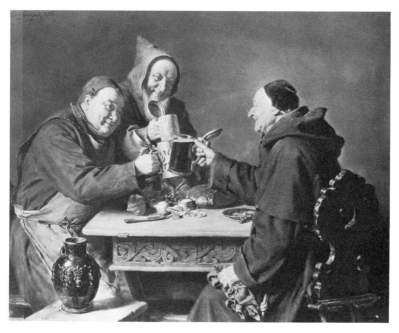

Alcohol has been widely used throughout history. Consumed unwisely, however, it can prove harmful and even deadly.

When a patient arrives unconscious in a hospital emergency room, one of the most likely causes is drug overdose, according to *Scientific American Medicine.* Often the overdose represents drug abuse or an attempted suicide. Indeed, of almost 49,000 reported alcohol poisonings in 1990, more than 21,000 were intentional, according to the American Association of Poison Control Centers. The study found that 79 of the poisonings resulted in death.

ETHYL ALCOHOL: FALSE ELIXIR OF LIFE

Anthropologists, the scientists who study the origin, development, and cultures of human civilization, believe that almost every prehistoric society that had access to fruit, honey, or starchy vegetables probably produced alcoholic beverages.

The key to making *ethyl alcohol*—the type of alcohol consumed as beer, wine, and liquor—is *fermentation*. In this process, yeast microorganisms attack sugars chemically and then transform them into carbon dioxide and alcohol. (This explains the ability of distillers to turn sugary fruits and honey into alcohol and also to use vegetables for this purpose, since the starch in vegetables is made up of sugar molecules.)

Ethyl alcohol—also called grain alcohol or ethanol—appears to have first been used by ancient societies in religious ceremonies and during social rites of passage, such as celebrations of birth, puberty, marriage, and the marking of a person's death. The Greeks and Romans accepted alcoholic intoxication as a normal occurrence on festive occasions.

In addition to ethyl alcohol, other common types of alcohol include *methyl alcohol*, also called methanol or wood alcohol, and *isopropyl alcohol*, also known as isopropanol or rubbing alcohol. These substances are highly poisonous to drink.

Although ethanol is also toxic, its effects are milder than those of either methanol or isopropanol, and in small or moderate amounts it can usually be imbibed safely. Even then, however, ethanol can influence the central nervous system, not only erasing an individual's normal social inhibitions but also affecting his or her judgment. In larger quantities, ethanol can be physically harmful and even deadly. The concentration of ethanol in American distilled spirits (e.g., gin, vodka, whiskey) varies from 40% to 50%. The ethanol concentration in wines ranges from 10% to 14%, and in most American beers it is about 4%.

The term *proof* on the container labels of distilled spirits refers to ethanol concentration. In the United States, the proof rating of an alcoholic beverage is equal to twice its ethanol concentration. Therefore, an 80-proof whiskey contains 40% alcohol.

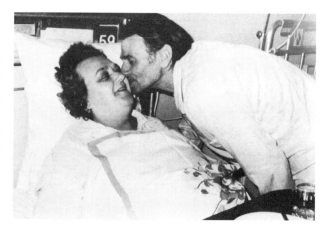

An Italian couple recovering after drinking wine containing a large concentration of poisonous methyl alcohol. In 1986, tainted wine killed a number of people in Italy.

Today, *alcohol abuse* is defined as frequent and excessive consumption of alcohol ("excessive" meaning to a point at which the alcohol causes clearly negative effects, such as loud or abusive behavior).

Alcohol, like sugar, is a simple food with limited nutritional value. Although it provides calories, it lacks proteins, minerals, and vitamins. Therefore, people who drink alcohol regularly while failing to eat properly commonly develop nutritional deficiencies.

In addition, ethanol activates substances in the liver that break down this drug. Low levels of ethanol activate the enzyme *alcohol dehydrogenase*, which rids the body of alcohol. High levels of ethanol, or long exposure to low levels, activates the protein *cytochrome P-450*, which breaks down ethanol. A resulting by-product of this breakdown is *acetaldehyde*, a substance that is harmful to the body but is usually itself quickly broken down. If, however, a person drinks too much ethanol too quickly, his or her body cannot break down acetaldehyde rapidly enough, and the toxic substance accumulates in the *hepatocytes* (liver cells).

Acetaldehyde interferes with various intercellular functions, preventing hepatocytes from producing certain proteins that the body needs and blocking the release of other proteins from liver cells. The buildup of proteins inside the cells causes the hepatocytes to expand. Moreover, the proteins attract water into the hepatocytes, further increasing the size of these cells.

The accumulation of swollen hepatocytes causes the liver to enlarge and inflicts serious damage on this organ. As liver cells are destroyed, they are replaced by abnormal connective tissue, which can eventually block blood flow into the liver. This condition, called *cirrhosis*, can ultimately prove fatal. Nevertheless, in many cases of cirrhosis, the liver may recover if the person stops abusing alcohol.

Alcohol has a more immediate influence on the central nervous system. It apparently interferes with the ability of impulses to travel from one nerve cell to the next and consequently depresses or hinders the functions of the nervous system. Alcohol goes to work first on those parts of the brain responsible for the most complex functions, such as thought, memory, and the smooth operation of muscles. Chronic alcohol abuse eventually causes sleep disturbances, bizarre behavior, memory loss, and brain damage.

Chronic alcohol abuse also interferes with the proper functioning of heart cells, apparently leading to *cardiomyopathy*, a disease in which the heart becomes enlarged and cannot function properly. Alcohol abuse may actually be the major cause of cardiomyopathy in the Western world.

Alcohol can take a particularly tragic toll on fetuses, causing *fetal alcohol syndrome (FAS)*. When a pregnant woman drinks, alcohol can reach her fetus by way of the *placenta*, the organ through which the fetus receives nourishment. Exposed to alcohol before birth, a child with FAS usually has an abnormally small brain and suffers from some degree of mental retardation. A short attention span, poor coordination, and behavioral problems can also result. Although it is not known precisely how alcohol harms the fetus, the drug apparently interferes with the multiplication of body cells that occurs during the fetus's development.

Despite this, it is difficult to know how much alcohol poses a danger to the fetus. Some pregnant women who drink heavily give birth to children with no signs of FAS, while some moderate drinkers produce infants who are affected. In addition, alcohol can increase the possibility of stillbirth and miscarriage. As a result, doctors advise pregnant women to avoid alcohol completely.

ACETYLSALICYLIC ACID

In mid-18th-century England, the Reverend Edmund Stone, writing a letter to a scientific society, described how he had found that the bark of the common white willow (*Salix alba vulgaris*) could cure the "agues" (fever). In 1829, the active ingredient in willow bark, called *salicin*, was purified for the first time, and its *antipyretic* (fever-reducing) power was demonstrated.

Salicin decomposes to yield both the sugar *glucose* and *salicylic alcohol*. In turn, salicylic alcohol can be converted into *salicylic acid*. A chemical variation of this latter substance, *sodium salicylate*, was first used to treat fevers in 1875.

Although an effective *analgesic* (pain-reducing) and antipyretic drug, sodium salicylate had an unfortunate side effect: it tended to cause stomach ulcers (open wounds in the wall of the stomach, which may bleed). However, the destructive acidic activity of salicylic acid was greatly reduced by combining it with *acetic anhydride* to produce *acetylsalicylic acid*. This compound was introduced at the end of the 19th century as aspirin.

About 20 billion aspirin tablets are sold each year in the United States. The drug's effectiveness is apparently due to its ability to inhibit the production of chemicals called *prostaglandins*, which are linked to inflammation. As with any drug, however, the more people who use aspirin, the greater the number of side effects that are observed.

Over the years, overdosage of aspirin has been blamed for many accidental poisonings in children and suicide deaths in adults. The number of such fatalities has fallen greatly during the past 20 years with the introduction of childproof caps on aspirin bottles, but aspirin poisoning as the result of abuse or sensitivity to the effects of acetylsalicylic acid continues to occur. In 1990, aspirin alone or in combination with other ingredients was responsible for more than 22,000 reported poisonings, according to the AAPCC. There were 42 aspirin-related deaths.

Acute acetylsalicylic acid poisoning stimulates the central nervous system, causing *hyperpnea*, or deep, rapid breathing. Through a complex series of physiological reactions, this eventually causes the concentration of acid in the blood to increase.

Tinnitus, or ringing in the ears, is probably the most common sign of aspirin poisoning. Other effects of acute poisoning include vomiting, hearing loss, and dizziness. The drug can also interfere with the body's ability to form blood clots. One reason for this is aspirin-induced liver damage. Since the liver produces *prothrombin*—an enzyme critical to the formation of blood clots (which stop the flow of blood through ruptured blood vessels)—damage to this organ may lead to excessive bleeding. At progressively higher doses, aspirin can cause delirium and respiratory failure, coma, and finally death.

In the early 1980s, medical experts began to warn that children suffering from chicken pox or influenza who take aspirin are at particular risk of developing *Reye's syndrome*, a rare, often fatal liver disease.

ACETAMINOPHEN: THE NONASPIRIN PAINKILLER

The nonaspirin pain reliever *acetaminophen* had been developed by 1893, although it did not become popular until 1949 and first became available without prescription in 1955. Its painkilling and fever-reducing effects are much the same as aspirin's.

Unlike aspirin, however, acetaminophen is only a weak inhibitor of prostaglandin synthesis, which may explain why it has much less of an anti-inflammatory effect than aspirin. Instead, acetaminophen seems to do its job by influencing the central nervous system, apparently by interfering with the activity of certain enzymes.

Acetaminophen is now an ingredient in more than 40% of commercially available analgesic products. Along with its increased use has come an increase in the number of cases of acetaminophen poisoning. According to the AAPCC's 1990 study, more than 104,000 acetaminophen-related poisonings (either with acetaminophen alone or in combination with other ingredients) were reported in 1990. Among these, 62 deaths occurred.

The toxicity of acetaminophen arises from its harmful effect on the liver. Normally, *glutathione*, a substance found in liver and other tissues, can *detoxify* acetaminophen or eliminate its poisonous quality. If too large a dose of acetaminophen has been ingested, however, there is not enough glutathione to detoxify the drug, leaving it free to damage liver cells. As in aspirin poisoning, liver damage caused by acetaminophen can reduce the amount of prothrombin produced by the organ, interfering with the body's ability to form blood clots. The body's ability to rapidly absorb acetaminophen from the intestines further enhances the toxicity of this drug.

COCAINE

Cocaine addiction is not new to the United States. An epidemic of abuse of this narcotic drug swept the United States from the late 19th century until the 1920s. The widespread use of cocaine was fueled by legal purchases of the drug in stores, through the mail, and in a variety of soft drinks and medicinal potions, some of which were used and praised by celebrities of the day.

The resulting increase in addiction to cocaine, and the subsequent popular association of the drug with crime, led to society's rejection of cocaine and the eventual move to make its possession illegal unless prescribed by a doctor.

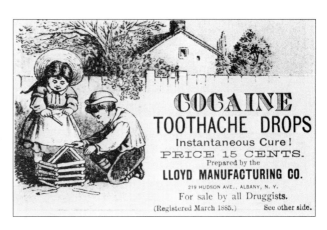

Although now illegal, cocaine was once a popular ingredient in soft drinks and medicines. As a result, an epidemic of cocaine abuse swept the United States from the late 19th century to the 1920s.

The current surge in cocaine abuse has taken a particularly harsh turn. The drug has swept into America's inner cities, where it has wrought havoc on families and neighborhoods. Cocaine has led to street shoot-outs as gangs fight over drug-dealing rights, to other kinds of crime, and to an increased number of babies born addicted to cocaine and mentally impaired because their mothers abused the drug during pregnancy.

Cocaine is an *alkaloid*, one of hundreds of substances produced by plants and made up of rings composed of carbon atoms combined with nitrogen. Alkaloids have *pharmacological activity*, that is, they affect the body in some way. Cocaine is produced by the *Erythroxylon coca* plant, which grows in Peru and Bolivia. For centuries, people in these countries have chewed the leaves of this plant, believing that it will increase their physical endurance and raise their sense of well-being.

Today, cocaine is chemically processed into various forms for use. It is commonly made into a *hydrochloride salt*, which physicians legally use as an anesthetic. In this application, cocaine is applied to the skin to reduce pain during medical procedures and works by blocking the transmission of nerve impulses.

When cocaine is taken to achieve a "high," the intensity and duration of its effects correspond to the rapidity with which the drug enters the bloodstream and how high its concentrations reach in the blood.

So-called *free-base cocaine*, also known as *rock* or *crack*, is created by mixing the hydrochloride salt of cocaine with ammonia or baking soda, thus freeing the drug from its salt form. In its free-base form, cocaine can be smoked in a tobacco cigarette or pipe. The inhaled drug is rapidly absorbed by the vast network of blood vessels in the lungs. From there, the drug travels in the blood directly to the heart and is then pumped through the rest of the body, including the brain. This movement of blood from the lungs to the brain takes only seconds, thereby contributing to the rapid, intense "high" obtained from using cocaine inhaled in this way as well as to the rapid onset of addiction to this narcotic.

Cocaine injected into the veins takes much longer to travel to the heart. Moreover, after reaching the heart it is first pumped to the lungs, then back to the heart, and finally to the rest of the body. This results in a greater delay before the drug reaches the brain. Cocaine takes even more time to reach the brain when it is taken by mouth or snorted through the nose.

Cocaine's Action on the Central Nervous System

Cocaine stimulates the so-called *reward system of the brain* (the system of nerve cells that, when stimulated, produces various types of emotions, including pleasure) by prolonging the activity of the neurotransmitter dopamine. After they have done their job of transmitting nerve signals—including signals in the reward center—dopamine and other neurotransmitters are normally either broken down or taken up

Crack cocaine, which can be smoked in a tobacco cigarette or pipe, is rapidly absorbed from the lungs into the bloodstream, causing a quick, intense "high." This also leads, however, to rapid cocaine addiction.

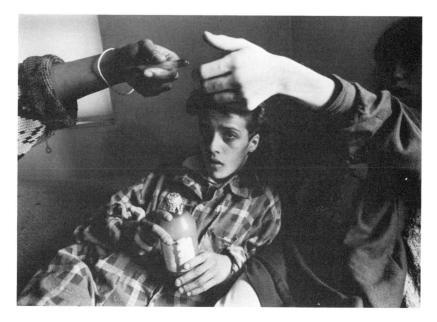

once again by the nerve that releases them. Cocaine blocks this re-uptake of dopamine by the nerves that typically release it and thus increases the stimulation of the reward center.

As a result, the immediate effects of cocaine can at first be deceptively pleasant. The drug can produce a sense of well-being, heightened awareness and drive, enhanced self-confidence, and sexual stimulation. This state may last for 30 to 90 minutes, but it is followed by a period of anxiety and depression that can last for hours.

Cocaine Poisoning

The sudden, severe effects of acute cocaine poisoning can result from a large dose of the drug. Because of their body chemistry, however, some people experience severe symptoms from even a small amount of cocaine. The symptoms of acute cocaine poisoning include headache, dizziness, blurred vision, and fainting; suicidal or violently aggressive behavior may follow. In more severe cases the victim lapses into a coma, and his or her respiratory system may fail, resulting in death.

Acute cocaine poisoning may also affect the *cardiovascular system* (heart and blood vessels), causing *thromboses* (blood clots that block the vessels) and *vasospasms* (tightening of the blood vessels so that blood flow is reduced; vasospasms can result in high blood pressure). Additionally, cocaine can cause *tachycardia* (abnormally rapid heartbeat) and *fibrillation* (very rapid contractions of small parts of the heart, without an overall strong contraction of the muscle. These effects prevent the heart from pumping blood effectively). Additionally, cocaine can cause *asystole*—a complete lack of contraction of the heart muscle. In fact, there have been numerous medical reports of *myocardial infarction* (heart attack) in young individuals who have used cocaine.

Moreover, the occurrence of vasospasm in the brain as a result of cocaine use can lead to what is termed *cerebrovascular accidents*, or *strokes*; in which blood flow to a particular part of the brain is disrupted, leading to the death of nerve cells in that area. A stroke can kill small areas of the brain, cause bleeding under the membranes surrounding the brain, and produce other severe problems that can lead to serious disability or death. Acute cocaine poisoning can also cause kidney failure and destruction of skeletal muscle.

Long-term cocaine use causes chronic poisoning, the symptoms of which include hallucinations and mental deterioration. In addition, cocaine reduces appetite to the extent that many chronic abusers of this drug become emaciated and suffer from vitamin deficiencies.

The increasing number of so-called cocaine babies is a particularly tragic consequence of cocaine abuse. As described earlier, cocaine taken during pregnancy reduces the supply of blood and oxygen that the mother provides to her fetus, retarding its growth and reducing its birth weight. Later, these children may suffer from a variety of problems, becoming sluggish and depressed or excitable and jittery.

The problem is especially severe in large cities such as New York, where crack smoking has reached epidemic proportions. The first crack babies entered kindergarten in 1990, and many showed learning difficulties, behavioral problems, and other effects from prenatal (before birth) cocaine exposure. This new wave of drug victims will pose enormous challenges to society's willingness and ability to serve them.

POLYCYCLIC ANTIDEPRESSANTS

The death of a loved one, divorce, loss of a job, and a long list of other personal tragedies commonly cause depression—depression that does not simply disappear with time and the well-meaning sympathy of friends. In fact, some cases of what is termed major depression are extremely difficult, if not impossible, to escape without medical treatment.

An individual suffering from major depression is plagued by intense sadness and despair, slowed mental processes, an inability to concentrate, pessimism, and a lack of self-esteem. A loss of energy, sexual drive, appetite, and weight also commonly occur.

Among the most widely used drugs in the treatment of major depression are imipramine, amitriptyline, desipramine, and other compounds known as *polycyclic antidepressants*. The term *polycyclic* refers to the fact that the molecular structure of these medications contains several rings or "cycles" of carbon atoms.

The polycyclic drugs enhance the effect of neurotransmitters in the brain, especially *norepinephrine* and *serotonin*. As with cocaine, polycyclic antidepressants interfere with the normal uptake of neurotransmitters, thus allowing them to continue to work. Eventually, however, this can "flood" the receptors on which these neurotransmitters operate, thus weakening their effect. The body may then make it difficult for neurotransmitters to send signals between nerve cells.

Because the polycyclic antidepressant drugs are very useful—they are often administered to treat suicidally depressed people—they are widely prescribed. Not surprisingly, then, they are a leading cause of serious drug overdose.

The symptoms of acute poisoning by polycyclic antidepressant drugs usually appear within a few hours of the ingestion of such a drug and include restlessness, *hypothermia* (abnormally low body temperature), and tachycardia. The victim may experience *hypotension* (abnormally low blood pressure) and slowed breathing and may lapse into a coma.

Chronic poisoning by a polycyclic antidepressant drug causes dryness of the mouth, drowsiness, abdominal pain, anxiety, inability to walk, blurred vision, hypotension, irregular heartbeat, liver damage, and convulsions.

BARBITURATES

Barbiturates, derivatives of a compound called *barbituric acid*, can depress the central nervous system. Their effects range from mild sedation (calming) to general anesthesia (the unconsciousness induced for surgery). They are dangerous if misused, however, and such misuse can lead to addiction and toxic overdose.

Barbiturates have been largely replaced by a family of drugs called *benzodiazepines*; nevertheless, barbiturate poisoning is still a major

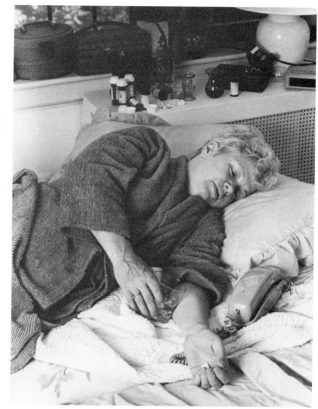

Although this photo is staged, it represents the dangers of barbiturate poisoning. Misuse of the drug, which depresses the central nervous system, can lead to death from respiratory failure.

problem in the United States. Death occurs in up to 12% of such cases. Most of these represent suicides, although accidental poisonings do occur among children and drug abusers.

The effects of moderate barbiturate intoxication resemble those caused by excessive alcohol consumption: sleepiness, mental confusion, and unsteadiness. In severe cases the victim can lapse into a coma, and his or her breathing may become either slow or rapid and shallow. Death can result from respiratory failure.

With overdose, the direct effect of a barbiturate, as well as the lack of oxygen caused by breathing problems, combine to inhibit the part of the brain called the *vasomotor center*. This area of the brain controls the diameter of blood vessels, increasing blood pressure by constricting (narrowing) the vessels, and lowering pressure by dilating (widening) them.

Because barbiturate poisoning causes the blood vessels to dilate and also causes the heart to pump less efficiently, the victim's blood pressure can fall very far below normal, resulting in shock. In combination with alcohol, the effects of barbiturates are especially severe.

Chronic barbiturate poisoning causes skin rash, mental confusion, difficulty in walking, dizziness, drowsiness, depression, irritability, and other disturbed behavior. The AAPCC cited more than 5,700 barbiturate poisonings in 1990, including 17 fatalities.

A POISONED WORLD?

A review of the hazards presented in this text might suggest that the world is truly a toxic place in which to live. Thus, for example, of the more than 1.7 million cases of poisoning reported in the 1990 study by the American Association of Poison Control Centers, only 171,017 were classified as suicide attempts or other forms of intentional misuse of toxic substances. Most were listed as accidental poisonings, indicating that the modern world does indeed present countless opportunities for unintended tragedy. But common sense and caution, exercised by individuals and by nations, can blunt many potential threats.

On an immediate level, a thorough respect for even nonprescription drugs is an effective weapon against overdose and abuse. On a global scale, the untold amounts of hazardous products released into the environment endanger the earth's ecology in general and human health in particular. Yet by understanding the long-range effects of previously overlooked poisons, humankind can better guard against damage from those that are already present in food, water, and soil, and can work to prevent the continued release of deadly substances into the environment.

APPENDIX:
FOR MORE INFORMATION

The following is a list of organizations that can provide further information about poisons and toxins.

American Association of Poison
   Control Centers
c/o Dr. Ted Tong
Health Sciences Center, Room 3204K
1501 North Campbell Hall
Tuscon, AZ 85725
(602) 626-7899

BioSciences Information Service
2100 Arch Street
Philadelphia, PA 19103
(215) 587-4800

Environmental Protection Agency
Public Information Center PM 211-13
401 M Street, Southwest
Washington, D.C. 20460
(202) 260-2080

Food and Drug Administration
Department of Health and Human
   Services
5600 Fishers Lane
Rockville, MD 20857

Institute for Scientific Information
3501 Market Street
Philadelphia, PA 19104
(215) 386-0100

International Society on Toxinology
c/o Dr. Philip Rosenberg

University of Connecticut School
   of Pharmacy
Storrs, CT 06268
(203) 486-2213

National Health Information Center
P.O. Box 1133
Washington, D.C. 20013
(800) 336-4797

National Institute for Occupational
   Safety and Health
300 Independence Avenue
Washington, D.C. 20201
Information Hotline: (800) 356-4674

National Institutes of Health
Public Inquiries
Building 31, Room 7A-32
9000 Rockville Pike
Bethesda, MD 20892

National Library of Medicine
8600 Rockville Pike
Bethesda, MD 20894
(301) 496-4000

Poison Prevention Week Council
P.O. Box 1543
Washington, D.C. 20013
(301) 504-0580

FURTHER READING

Bergin, Edward, and Ronald E. Grandon. *The American Survival Guide: How to Survive in Your Toxic Environment.* New York: Avon, 1984.

Brookes, Vincent J. *Poisons: Properties, Chemical Identification, Symptoms, and Emergency Treatment.* Melbourne, FL: Robert E. Kreiger, 1975.

Bucherl, Wolfgang, et al., eds. *Venomous Animals and Their Venoms.* San Diego, CA: Harcourt Brace Jovanovich, 1968.

Chlad, Dorothy. *Poisons Make You Sick.* Chicago: Children's Press, 1984.

Cooper, M. G. *Risk: Man-Made Hazards to Man.* New York: Oxford University Press, 1985.

Devries, A., and E. Kochva. *Toxins of Animal and Plant Origin.* New York: Gordon and Breach, 1973.

Dreisbach, Robert H., and William O. Robertson. *Handbook of Poisoning: Prevention, Diagnosis, & Treatment.* Norwalk, CT: Appleton & Lange, 1987.

Environmental Protection Agency Staff. *Toxicology Handbook.* Rockville, MD: Government Institutions, 1986.

Gilman, Alfred Goodman, et al., eds. *The Pharmacological Basis of Therapeutics.* 7th ed. New York: Macmillan, 1985.

Goodman, Sondra, et al. *Guide to Hazardous Products Around the Home.* 2nd ed. Springfield, MO: Household Hazardous Waste Project, Southwest Missouri State University's Office of Continuing Education, 1989.

Habermehl, G. *Venomous Animals and Their Toxins.* New York: Springer-Verlag, 1981.

Halstead, Bruce W. *Poisonous and Venomous Marine Animals of the World.* Princeton, NJ: Darwin Press, 1988.

Hardegree, M. Carolyn, and Anthony T. Tu, eds. *Handbook of Natural Toxins.* New York: Marcel Dekker, 1988.

Hardin, James W., and Jay M. Arena. *Human Poisoning from Native and Cultivated Plants.* 2nd ed. Durham, NC: Duke University Press, 1974.

Harding, Keith A., and Kenneth R. Welch. *Poisonous Snakes of the World: A Checklist.* Elmsford, NY: Pergamon Books, 1980.

Harris, John B. *Natural Toxins: Animal, Plant, and Microbial.* New York: Oxford University Press, 1987.

James, Wilma R. *Know Your Poisonous Plants.* Happy Camp, CA: Nature-graph Publications, 1973.

Kinghorn, Douglas A. *Toxic Plants.* New York: Columbia University Press, 1979.

Kirsch, Catherine A. *Things that Sting.* Lorain, OH: Dayton Laboratories, 1978.

Lampe, Kenneth F., and Mary A. McCann. *The AMA Handbook of Poisonous and Injurious Plants.* Chicago: American Medical Association, 1985.

Landrigan, Philip J., and Irving J. Selikoff, eds. *Occupational Health in the 1990's: Developing a Platform for Disease Prevention, Annals of the New York Academy of Sciences,* vol. 572. New York: New York Academy of Sciences, 1989.

Mattison, Christopher. *Snakes of the World.* New York: Facts on File, 1984.

Milligan, Jacquie. *Spring Cleaning: Household Poisons.* Minneapolis: Denison & Co., 1986.

Minton, Sherman A., and Madge Rutherford Minton. *Venomous Reptiles.* New York: Scribners, 1980.

Pater, A. R., M. Roy and G. M. Wilson. "Self-Poisoning and Alcohol." *Lancet.* 787 (1972): 1099–102.

Russell, Findlay E. *Marine Toxins and Venomous and Poisonous Marine Animals.* Neptune City, NJ: T.F.H. Publications, 1971.

Schroeder, Henry A. *The Poisons Around Us.* New Canaan, CT: Keats, 1978.

Schultes, Richard Evans, and Albert Hoffman. *Plants of the Gods: Origins of Hallucinogenic Use.* New York: McGraw-Hill, 1979.

Simon, Seymour. *Poisonous Snakes.* New York: Macmillan, 1981.

GLOSSARY

acetaminophen a nonaspirin pain reliever

acute poisoning toxic exposure causing severe effects in a short amount of time

alkaloid a bitter-tasting plant product that can be used as a drug; common alkaloids include caffeine, nicotine, and morphine

anaerobic able to survive without oxygen

analgesic a pain-reducing drug

anaphylaxis an immediate and often lethal allergic reaction to venom or some other foreign substance, caused by a previous exposure to that substance

anatoxin a poison found in mushrooms that damages the membrane and nucleus of cells

antibody a naturally occurring, disease-fighting agent

antidote a substance that counteracts the effects of poisons

antivenin a mixture of antibodies used to treat the toxic effects of a venom

apnea temporary stoppage of breathing

asbestos a fibrous, toxic mineral once widely used in construction and industry

asbestosis inflammation of and damage to the lungs caused by the inhalation of asbestos particles; the main symptom is dyspnea

asystole a condition in which the heart muscle stops contracting

ataxia lack of motor coordination

atropine a toxin that interferes with neurotransmitters and damages the nervous system

barbiturate a drug that causes depression of the central nervous system

botulism a type of food intoxication related to the ingestion of the bacterium *Clostridium botulinum* and characterized by muscle weakness, paralysis, and, often, death

bronchospasm rapid contraction and relaxation of the air passages leading to the lungs

cardiotoxic poisonous to the heart

cardiovascular system the heart and blood vessels

caustic a burning or corrosive quality that can damage living tissue

central nervous system the brain and spinal cord

cholera a gastrointestinal disease caused by the bacterium *Vibrio cholerae*

chorea a nervous disorder characterized by erratic, rapid body movements

chronic poisoning poisoning occurring through repeated exposure to a substance over an extended period of time

ciguatoxin a neurotoxin found in some saltwater fish that causes a food-borne disease when consumed by humans; its effects include numbness, paralysis, and occasionally death; it is unaffected by heating, freezing, or storage

cirrhosis a disease caused by alcohol abuse and characterized by the growth of abnormal tissue that blocks the flow of blood to the liver

constipation a condition in which bowel movements are infrequent or incomplete

contamination the presence of harmful substances, including infectious organisms, that make a food or beverage unfit to consume

convulsion a violent series of involuntary muscle contractions in the face, torso, or limbs

cyanosis oxygen deficiency in the blood, marked by a bluish discoloration of the skin

cytotoxin a toxin exercising a harmful effect on the cells of specific organs

defoliant a chemical used to remove foliage from growing plants

delirium a condition of extreme mental excitement characterized by faulty perception, loss of memory, a rapid succession of confused and unconnected ideas, and often accompanied by illusions and hallucinations

detoxify eliminate poisonous qualities

dinoflagellate a tiny, plantlike microorganism; it produces a neurotoxin that can cause severe food intoxication after the ingestion of contaminated food

dysentery a disease caused by bacteria and resulting in severe diarrhea; it deprives the body of essential nutrients

dyspnea shortness of breath; difficulty in breathing

electrolyte a substance that contributes to the maintenance of normal conditions inside the body, especially in the blood, and takes on an electrical charge when dissolved in solution

Enterobacteriaceae a family of bacteria found in water, which often dwells in the large intestines of vertebrates and can cause intestinal diseases

enterotoxigenic term that refers to bacteria that produce toxins in the intestines

enzymes proteins that induce chemical reactions in the body without being changed themselves

fibrillation rapid contraction of small parts of the heart without an overall, rhythmic contraction of the heart muscle; it prevents the heart from effectively pumping blood

food intoxication food-borne disease caused by a toxin rather than directly by a microorganism

food poisoning food-borne disease caused by a microorganism

fungicide a chemical that kills fungi, such as molds

gastric lavage a method of removing poisons from the stomach; emptying and "washing out" the stomach through a tube inserted down the throat

gastroenteritis inflammation of the stomach and lining of the gastrointestinal tract

hemodialysis a technique that removes waste products from the blood of people with kidney failure

hemoglobin a protein in red blood cells that carries oxygen from the lungs to the tissues

hemotoxin a poison affecting the circulatory system, causing blood clots, internal bleeding, low blood pressure, and shock

hyperpnea deep, rapid breathing

hypothermia abnormally low body temperature

incubation period the interval between the body's infection by an organism and the manifestation of the infection's first symptoms; the period in which an infection is not recognizable

intoxication the process of poisoning

jaundice yellowing of the skin due to the excessive accumulation of the pigment bilirubin in the blood

mesothelioma a type of cancer caused by exposure to asbestos

nematocysts tiny stinging organs located on the tentacles of jellyfish and related organisms; nematocysts release a poison that can cause failure of the circulatory system

neurologic related to the nervous system

neurotoxin a substance that poisons or destroys nerve tissue

neurotransmitter a chemical substance that carries impulses from one nerve to another

paresthesia an abnormal sensation, such as burning or tingling

pasteurization the process of eliminating living microorganisms from milk, wines, fruit juices, or other beverages by heating and then quickly chilling the beverage

pathogenic capable of causing disease

pesticide a substance used to destroy pests

poison any substance that, once inside the body, produces chemical reactions that interfere with normal bodily functions

respiratory paralysis failure of the muscles that control breathing

salmonellosis a form of gastroenteritis caused by bacteria of the genus *Salmonella*

solvents substances in which other materials can be dissolved

spasms sudden, involuntary muscle contractions

stroke disruption of the blood flow to a particular part of the brain, causing the death of the nerve cells in that area; it can lead to serious disability or death

syrup of ipecac a poison-control product that induces vomiting

tachycardia an abnormally rapid heartbeat

thrombosis a blood clot that blocks vessels and hinders the flow of blood

tourniquet a device, such as a cloth bandage encircling a limb, that stops the flow of blood through a large artery

toxicity the degree to which a substance is poisonous

toxin a poisonous substance produced by a plant or animal

uremia an excess of waste products in the blood that comes from the kidney's inability to produce urine

vasomotor center part of the brain that controls the diameter of blood vessels

vasospasm a contraction of blood vessels that reduces the flow of blood through the body

venom poison excreted by animals and passed on to victims through bites or stings

INDEX

PICTURE CREDITS

Marc Kusinitz holds a doctorate in biology from New York University and has been a science writer for over 10 years. He was news editor at the *New York State Journal of Medicine* and editor of *New Medical Science*. His articles have appeared in the *New York Times*, the *San Jose Mercury News*, and *Technology Review*. He is an author of Chelsea House volumes in both THE ENCYCLOPEDIA OF PSYCHOACTIVE DRUGS and THE ENCYCLOPEDIA OF HEALTH series. Formerly the science writer at the Public Affairs Department of the University of Maine, Orono, Dr. Kusinitz is now assistant director for media relations at the Johns Hopkins Medical Institutions in Baltimore, Maryland.

Dale C. Garell, M.D., is medical director of California Children Services, Department of Health Services, County of Los Angeles. He is also associate dean for curriculum at the University of Southern California School of Medicine and clinical professor in the Department of Pediatrics & Family Medicine at the University of Southern California School of Medicine. From 1963 to 1974, he was medical director of the Division of Adolescent Medicine at Children's Hospital in Los Angeles. Dr. Garell has served as president of the Society for Adolescent Medicine, chairman of the youth committee of the American Academy of Pediatrics, and as a forum member of the White House Conference on Children (1970) and White House Conference on Youth (1971). He has also been a member of the editorial board of the *American Journal of Diseases of Children.*

C. Everett Koop, M.D., Sc.D., is former Surgeon General, deputy assistant secretary for health, and director of the Office of International Health of the U.S. Public Health Service. A pediatric surgeon with an international reputation, he was previously surgeon-in-chief of Children's Hospital of Philadelphia and professor of pediatric surgery and pediatrics at the University of Pennsylvania. Dr. Koop is the author of more than 175 articles and books on the practice of medicine. He has served as surgery editor of the *Journal of Clinical Pediatrics* and editor-in-chief of the *Journal of Pediatric Surgery*. Dr. Koop has received nine honorary degrees and numerous other awards, including the Denis Brown Gold Medal of the British Association of Paediatric Surgeons, the William E. Ladd Gold Medal of the American Academy of Pediatrics, and the Copernicus Medal of the Surgical Society of Poland. He is a chevalier of the French Legion of Honor and a member of the Royal College of Surgeons, London.